In the Fullness of Time

In the Fullness of Time

*Recovery from Borderline
Personality Disorder*

MARY C. ZANARINI

OXFORD
UNIVERSITY PRESS

Oxford University Press is a department of the University of Oxford. It furthers
the University's objective of excellence in research, scholarship, and education
by publishing worldwide. Oxford is a registered trade mark of Oxford University
Press in the UK and certain other countries.

Published in the United States of America by Oxford University Press
198 Madison Avenue, New York, NY 10016, United States of America.

CIP data is on file at the Library of Congress
ISBN 978-0-19-537060-7

9 8 7 6 5 4 3 2 1

Printed by Sheridan Books, Inc., United States of America

For Frances Frankenburg

To whom I owe a debt of gratitude that I will never be able to repay

CONTENTS

1. History of the Borderline Diagnosis   1

2. Models of the Core Features of Borderline Personality Disorder   7

3. Earlier Studies of the Longitudinal Course of BPD   21

4. The McLean Study of Adult Development (MSAD)   35

5. The Symptoms of Borderline Personality Disorder Assessed in
    MSAD   45

6. The Long-Term Course of the Symptoms of Borderline Personality
    Disorder   67

7. Symptomatic Remissions and Recurrences of the Borderline
    Diagnosis   81

8. Prevalence and Predictors of Physically Self-Destructive Acts over
    Time   87

9. Additional Symptom Areas over Time   99

10. Psychosocial Functioning over Time   107

11. Recovery from Borderline Personality Disorder   117

12. Predictors of Time-to-Remission and Recovery   129

13. Co-occurring Disorders over Time   141

14. Mental Health Treatment over Time   149

15. Physical Health and Medical Treatment   161

16. Adult Victimization over Time   171

17. Sexual Issues over Time   175

18. Defense Mechanisms over Time   181

19. Going Forward   189

REFERENCES   193
ABOUT THE AUTHOR   209
INDEX   211

In the Fullness of Time

History of the Borderline Diagnosis

Borderline personality disorder (BPD) is a common psychiatric disorder; the best epidemiological evidence estimating that about 2% of American adults meet *Diagnostic and Statistical Manual of Mental Disorders* (*DSM*) criteria for BPD (Lenzenweger, Lane, Loranger, & Kessler, 2007; Swartz, Blazer, George, & Winfield, 1990; Trull, Jahng, Tomko, Wood, & Sher, 2010). It has also been estimated that approximately 19% of psychiatric inpatients and approximately 11% of psychiatric outpatients meet criteria for BPD (Widiger & Frances, 1989). In addition, cross-sectional studies have found that BPD is associated with high levels of mental health service utilization (Bender et al., 2001) and a serious degree of psychosocial impairment (Skodol et al., 2002).

However, BPD still has not gained wide use in many clinical settings. Much of this reluctance to give the borderline diagnosis is due to stigma. Many mental health professionals believe that the borderline diagnosis is pejorative, indicating a patient who is difficult to handle and has a poor prognosis. Clinical experience suggests that treating those with BPD can be challenging but can be done with success by providers in the community. In addition, the belief that those with BPD have a poor prognosis is based on outdated information and contradicts the findings of two recent longitudinal studies (Gunderson, Stout, et al., 2011; Zanarini, Frankenburg, Reich, & Fitzmaurice, 2012). In fact, it has been found that BPD has the best symptomatic prognosis of any of the major psychiatric illnesses.

A second reason for its lack of use is that BPD is one of our newer psychiatric diagnoses. It only entered our official nomenclature in 1980 (*DSM-III*; American Psychiatric Association, 1980). In addition, it is important to note that it grew more out of the psychoanalytic tradition than the tradition of descriptive psychiatry. This fact may have made it difficult for many clinicians to adopt the borderline diagnosis, as they viewed psychodynamic thought as old-fashioned and out of step with the needs of modern mental health professionals. Following is a brief history of the borderline diagnosis, beginning with the work of Adolph Stern and ending with the forerunner of our current nomenclature—*DSM-IV/5*.

Adolph Stern (1938) was the first author to write about the "borderline" patient. He described a disorder that was between neurosis and psychosis—the two large divisions of psychopathology that were recognized by analysts and general psychiatrists at that time (Stone, 1990). Stern believed that such patients exhibited symptoms of a neurotic nature and symptoms of a psychotic nature—the latter category being far larger than it is today.

Stern noted several key features of this condition. The first of these features is having narcissistic character traits, which Stern attributed to early childhood adversity—from which arises an affective (narcissistic) "malnutrition." The second of these features is "psychic bleeding." Stern describes this feature as a complete collapse into inactivity when faced with stress or danger. The third of these features is inordinate hypersensitivity. Stern sees this feature as a way to identify danger in the interpersonal realm. However, it leads to being easily offended by comments of others that have no malevolent intent. The fourth feature is psychic rigidity or constant watchful waiting for danger. The fifth feature is negative therapeutic reactions. By this, Stern means a regressive reaction to comments by the therapist that includes anger, feelings of depression, suicidal ideation, and an ever-increasing dependency on the therapist who made the poorly received comment. The sixth feature is feelings of inferiority that are both unrealistic and used to remain in a passive role, particularly in relationship to their therapist. The seventh feature is masochism; or, in the words of Stern, feelings of "self-pity." The eighth feature is "somatic" insecurity or anxiety. This symptom cluster refers to a tendency to become very anxious when faced with a defeat, which activates the system of chronic feelings of inferiority; or, in other words, a tendency to react in an "all or none" manner. The ninth feature is the use of projective defenses, which is described as a tendency to unrealistically view the environment as dangerous. The tenth feature is difficulties in reality-testing, which are described as a childlike idealization of the analyst. Stern recommends a supportive approach to these patients, at least initially.

A number of other psychoanalysts used other terms for these basically non-psychotic patients. Deutsch (1942) referred to "as if" patients who lacked a core identity, while Zetzel (1968) coined the term the "so-called good hysteric" to describe patients who were more fragile than they first appeared to be. Schimdeberg (1947) referred to their often chaotic behavior and varied symptoms as "stably unstable."

Other investigators linked these "borderline" patients to schizophrenia. Zilboorg (1941) referred to them as "ambulatory schizophrenia," while Hoch and Polatin (1949) referred to them as "pseudoneurotic schizophrenia." Knight (1953) took an intermediate position about the relationship of these patients to psychosis. He referred to "borderline states" and stressed the fluidity of the psychopathology of these patients when in unstructured situations.

Frosch (1960) focused on their cognitive functioning, particularly their relationship to reality, their feeling of reality, and their ability to test reality consistently. He used the term "psychotic character" to describe these patients. By "relationship to reality," he meant hallucinations and illusions that are transient and reversible. By "feeling of reality," he meant experiences of depersonalization and other forms of dissociation. By "reality testing," he meant the ability to detect shared reality without much effort.

However, it is primarily the work of Kernberg (1967) from the 1960s and Gunderson from the 1970s (Gunderson & Singer, 1975) that has shaped the criteria for BPD in *DSM-III (American Psychiatric Association, 1980), DSM-III-R (American Psychiatric Association, 1987)*, and *DSM-IV/ 5 (which use the same criteria for BPD) (American Psychiatric Association, 1994 and 2013)*. Kernberg presented a careful and very detailed description of a level of psychopathology that he called *borderline personality organization* (BPO), which was set between psychotic personality and neurotic personality organization. BPO was defined by problems in four areas. The first was a tendency to exhibit symptoms in a variety of areas, such as anxiety, polysymptomtic neuroses, and a lower level personality disorder, such as narcissistic or antisocial personality disorder. The second was reliance on a number of lower level defense mechanisms: splitting, primitive idealization, denial, projective identification, omnipotence, and devaluation. The third was internal object relations marked by the inability to integrate positive and negative aspects of the self and others so that one's view of oneself and others was more nuanced and more realistic. The fourth was a history of extreme frustrations and aggression toward others. In this regard, Kernberg was unsure if the excessive aggression is due to actual frustrations or is constitutional in nature.

Gunderson and Singer published an important literature review in 1975 (Gunderson & Singer, 1975). From this review, they extracted six features that they believed defined what they called *BPD*. The first of these features was the presence of intense affect, typically of an angry or depressive nature. The second of these features was a history of impulsivity. Here both self-mutilation and suicide attempts were listed, as were promiscuity and substance abuse. The third of these features was apparent social adaptiveness in both the social and vocational realms. The fourth feature was brief psychotic experiences, which tended to be of a paranoid nature and to appear in unstructured situations. The fifth of these features was psychological testing performance, which was marked by a good performance on structured tests, such as the Wechsler Adult Intelligence Scale (WAIS), and more overly delineated responses on unstructured tests, such as the Rorschach. The sixth feature was interpersonal relationships marked by intensity and marred by manipulation, devaluation, and demandingness.

PLACE IN PSYCHIATRIC NOMENCLATURE

With the publication of *DSM-III*, BPD was no longer linked in our nomenclature as a subthreshold or developing form of schizophrenia. Rather, the work of Spitzer and colleagues separated BPD, which had no cognitive criteria, from schizotypal personality disorder, which was marked by oddities of thought and behavior (Spitzer, Endicott, & Gibbon, 1979).

However, BPD was still not viewed as a separate and distinct disorder by many clinical observers, but tended to be seen as part of a series of spectrum of disorders that arose, in turn, over the years to capture the attention of mental health professionals. The first of these conceptualizations, which organized much of clinical care and empirical research in the 1980s, focused on the chronic dysphoria and affective lability of borderline patients. In this view, borderline personality was thought of as being an affective spectrum disorder (Akiskal, 1981; Stone, 1980).

Both the second and third of the more recent theories of borderline psychopathology have arisen during the 1990s. Links and his associates have proposed that BPD is best conceptualized as an impulse spectrum disorder (i.e., a disorder related to substance use disorders, antisocial personality disorder, and perhaps eating disorders) (Links, Heslegrave, & van Reekum, 1999). In this view, BPD is not seen as an attenuated or atypical form of one of these impulse spectrum disorders. Rather, these authors suggest that BPD is a specific form of psychiatric disorder that may share a propensity to action with other disorders of impulse dyscontrol.

At about the same time, Herman and van der Kolk (1987) suggested that BPD might better be conceptualized as a chronic form of post-traumatic stress disorder (PTSD). This theoretical observation led, in part, to the view that BPD is a trauma spectrum disorder, related to PTSD and dissociative disorders, including dissociative identity disorder.

At the present time, BPD is viewed by most experts in the field as a specific disorder that is valid according to the criteria outlined by Robins and Guze (1970) over 45 years ago. More specifically, research has shown that BPD has a characteristic clinical presentation that can be distinguished from that of other disorders (Zanarini, Gunderson, Frankenburg, & Chauncey, 1990), something of its etiology (both environmental and biological factors) is known (Torgersen et al., 2000; Zanarini et al., 1997), it "runs" in families (Gunderson, Zanarini, et al., 2011), and the course of the disorder is being mapped out in ever increasing detail (Gunderson, Stout, et al., 2011; Zanarini, Frankenburg, Reich, & Fitzmaurice, 2012).

However, patients with BPD are often treated by clinicians, particularly pharmacotherapists, as though they had some type of bipolar disorder. They are also treated by a substantial number of clinicians, particularly psychotherapists, as if their childhood adversity were the sole cause of their distress and disability. But neither of these viewpoints helps us to understand the essential nature of BPD. The fact that many clinicians mistake the hair-trigger lability of borderline patients for the sustained mood swings of bipolar disorder hides rather than illuminates the core problem or problems with which borderline patients struggle. In a like manner, viewing borderline patients solely as victims of the brutality or negligence of others ignores the strong sense of agency that is characteristic of many borderline patients and an important aspect of their will to get well.

Currently, there are several models of borderline psychopathology. Each points to different features of the disorder as core to defining it and understanding it. The next chapter will describe these models, with most emphasis on the model of BPD that has grown out of our research and clinical work with these troubled but challenging and worthwhile people.

2

Models of the Core Features
of Borderline Personality Disorder

A number of models of borderline psychopathology have been suggested by leading theorists in the field. Linehan has suggested that BPD is best understood as a disorder of emotional dysregulation (1993). In this model, the quick reactivity of borderline patients (and the lack of strategies to handle this deficit) is the core feature of BPD. Gunderson has suggested that BPD is best understood as a disorder of attachment (1984). In this model, fear of aloneness and abandonment are the core conflicts with which patients with BPD suffer and are the most salient features of the disorder.

These two models are different in their emphasis on different areas of phenomenology (affective and interpersonal symptoms, respectively) as the primary problem of borderline patients. They also frame these problems differently, with Linehan suggesting a deficit model and Gunderson suggesting a conflict model. These models are alike in that they see the other symptoms of BPD as secondary in nature and reactive to the primary feature, a means of coping with it, or some combination of the two.

TRIPARTITE MODEL OF THE ETIOLOGY OF BPD

About 20 years ago, our group proposed a tripartite model of the etiology of BPD (Zanarini & Frankenburg, 1997). We suggested that three interlocking factors were necessary for the development of BPD. The first of these factors was a childhood environment that was traumatic. These experiences of childhood adversity were thought to engender intense feelings of sorrow, rage, shame, and/or terror. The second of these factors was a vulnerable or "hyperbolic" temperament (Zanarini & Frankenburg, 1994). By "hyperbolic temperament," we meant a tendency to easily take offense and to try to manage the resulting sense of perpetual umbrage by persistently insisting that others pay attention to the enormity of one's inner pain. However, these unremitting attempts to get comfort and support are usually indirect and involve a covert reproach of the listener's "insensitivity," "stupidity," or "malevolence." The third of these factors was a "triggering" event or series of events, which could be either normative or traumatic. These triggering events were also thought to have usually occurred either in late adolescence or early adulthood. Without such an event or series of events, a potentially borderline person might be viewed as intense and demanding but not clearly ill or impaired. However, the presence of such a triggering event acted as the catalyst for the fruition of a full-blown case of BPD with its characteristic symptom pattern.

COMPLEX MODEL OF BORDERLINE PSYCHOPATHOLOGY

We have more recently proposed what we term a "complex" model of borderline psychopathology (Zanarini, Frankenburg, Hennen, Reich, & Silk, 2005). In this model, as in our prior model, borderline patients typically have what we have termed a "hyperbolic" temperament (Zanarini & Frankenburg, 1994). However, BPD would not emerge without some type of kindling event or events. These events can be normative, such as taking one's first job or beginning one's first intimate relationship. They can also be traumatic in nature. These kindling events can have first occurred in early childhood or latency. They can also have first occurred in early, middle, or late adolescence, or adulthood. In any case, the severity of the kindling event or series of events is associated with the severity of the resulting borderline psychopathology. In fact, the severity of the temperamental vulnerability seems to interact with the severity of the kindling event or events to determine the overall severity of borderline psychopathology.

As the result of the interactions of a vulnerable or hyperbolic temperament and kindling events, the symptoms of BPD emerge. Some of these symptoms are acute and others are temperamental (Zanarini, Frankenburg, Hennen, & Silk, 2003).

This model differs from our earlier tripartite model in a number of important ways. First, we now place the most emphasis on an inborn vulnerable or hyperbolic temperament rather than on adverse or traumatic childhood experiences. Second, we now highlight that kindling experiences can occur at any age, and thus, the onset of BPD may be in childhood or early to mid-adolescence as well as late adolescence or young adulthood. Third, we now believe that the severity of a potentially borderline person's temperamental vulnerability interacts with the severity of their kindling experiences to determine the overall severity of their borderline psychopathology. In our prior model, there was an assumption that most borderline patients had endured serious pathological childhood experiences, and as a result, most cases of BPD were severe.

CONTINUUM OF BORDERLINE PSYCHOPATHOLOGY

Clinical experience suggests, however, that there is a continuum of borderline psychopathology. All patients we would consider "borderline" meet rigorous criteria for the disorder. In fact, we have found that outpatient borderlines and symptomatic volunteers (who may or may not have a history of psychiatric treatment) typically manifest borderline psychopathology that is equal in severity to that of inpatients with BPD (e.g., Zanarini, Frankenburg, & Parachini, 2004). All patients we would consider borderline are also in tremendous inner pain but unfortunately handle this pain in an awkward and self-defeating manner (Zanarini & Frankenburg, 1994).

However, four factors distinguish mild from more severe cases of BPD. The first factor is the number of co-occurring Axis I disorders from which they suffer. We have found that those with milder cases of BPD tend to have fewer co-occurring disorders than those with more severe cases, and that those with milder cases tend, in particular, to be less likely to meet criteria for an anxiety disorder (e.g., Zanarini, Frankenburg, & Parachini, 2004).

Another factor is the degree of their psychosocial impairment. This impairment can be relatively mild, or it can be quite severe. Some borderline patients work or go to school successfully and have active social lives as well. Others support themselves on disability payments and live quite isolated lives. Some have supportive relationships with their family of origin, and others have cut off contact with their parents and siblings. How much of this impairment is due to natural endowment and how much is due to the reaction of important others, including treating clinicians and protective family members, is an open question.

A third factor is the strength of their will to get better. Some borderline patients have a strong fighting spirit, but others have such a strong need to have their inner pain affirmed or such severe experiential avoidance (of anxiety-provoking experiences) that they gradually slide into the role of chronic patient.

The fourth factor is their ability to use treatment to help themselves. Some borderline patients are able to use psychotherapy to gain traction in their lives, yet others are unable to use treatment effectively and in fact, seem to have a toxic reaction to it. In many ways, these differences can be summed up as some borderline patients have a sense of agency and hopefulness about the future, while in contrast, others have a firm belief (or hope) that the rules of life do not apply to them because of what has happened to them.

KEY FEATURES OF BORDERLINE PERSONALITY DISORDER

We believe that there are two key features of BPD. The first of these features is the intense inner pain that they live with on a chronic basis. This pain is distinguished from the pain of others by its multifaceted nature and its overall amplitude (Zanarini, Frankenburg, DeLuca, et al., 1998). It consists of both dysphoric affects (e.g., I feel grief-stricken, I feel completely panicked) and dysphoric cognitions (e.g., like I'm being tortured, damaged beyond repair) that are quite specific to BPD. More recently, another group (Zittel, Conklin, & Westen, 2005) has also found that severe inner pain is both characteristic and distinguishing for borderline patients.

The second feature, which is perhaps better known to clinicians, is the awkward nature of the efforts that borderline patients make to handle this pain and to express it. Some of these efforts are behavioral or impulsive in nature. The most troubling impulsive action patterns are self-mutilation and help-seeking suicide threats and gestures. Other efforts to obtain needed comfort and support are interpersonal in nature. They include such maladaptive patterns such as devaluation and demandingness. While the impulsive acts tend to frighten clinicians, these interpersonal patterns tend to anger them. In fact, inexperienced clinicians often think of them as forms of misbehavior. We think it is less pejorative and more accurate to describe them as "outmoded survival strategies." In other words, these are interpersonal patterns that were used when they were younger that helped in some way to lessen their pain.

Two key questions emerge. First, what caused the intense inner pain of borderline patients? Second, why do they handle it in such a self-defeating manner? In terms of the first question, we had assumed about two decades ago that only serious adversity would have resulted in the intense inner pain that both characterizes and distinguishes borderline patients from those in other diagnostic groups (Zanarini, Frankenburg, & DeLuca, 1998). We now believe that many borderline patients are so temperamentally vulnerable that much more subtle experiences can engender the suffering that they both insist that others pay attention to and of which they are so ashamed.

ENVIRONMENTAL FACTORS OF ETIOLOGICAL SIGNIFICANCE

Of course, a related question arises: What is serious and what is mild adversity? The early psychoanalytic theories of the etiology of BPD focused on subtle difficulties in intrapsychic development that occurred during the first years of life.

Psychoanalytic Theories of the Pathogenesis of BPD

In the first of these theories, which we have reviewed earlier, Kernberg (1967) suggested that excessive early aggression leads the young child to split her positive and negative images of herself and her mother. This excess aggression may be inborn, or it may have been caused by real frustrations. In either case, the pre-borderline child is unable to merge her positive and negative images and attendant affects to achieve a more realistic and ambivalent view of herself and others.

In the second of these theories, Adler and Buie (1979) suggested that failures in early mothering lead to a failure to develop stable object constancy. Because the pre-borderline child's mothering was inconsistent and oftentimes insensitive and nonempathic, the child fails to develop a consistent view of herself or others that she can use in times of stress to comfort and sustain herself.

In the third of these theories, Masterson (1972) suggested that fear of abandonment is the central factor in borderline psychopathology. He believes that the mother of the future borderline patient interfered with her child's natural autonomous strivings by withdrawing emotionally when the child acted in an independent manner during the phase of development that Mahler (1971) has termed "separation-individuation." Later experiences that require independent behavior lead to a recrudescence of the dysphoria and abandonment panic that the borderline patient felt as a child when faced with a seemingly insoluble dilemma (either continue to behave dependently, or lose needed emotional support).

Empirical Investigations of Environmental Factors

Five environmental factors thought to be of etiological importance have been the subject of extensive empirical investigation. These kindling factors are: (1) early separations and losses, (2) disturbed parental involvement, (3) experiences of verbal and emotional abuse, (4) experiences of physical and sexual abuse, and (5) experiences of physical and emotional neglect.

Investigations of early separations and losses and disturbed parental involvement were undertaken to assess the accuracy of the psychoanalytic theories described earlier in this chapter. The later studies of abuse and neglect arose from clinical observations that many borderline patients, particularly inpatients with BPD, reported having had more extreme experiences of childhood adversity.

STUDIES OF EARLY SEPARATIONS AND LOSSES

Most studies of prolonged early separations and losses have found that they are common in the childhood histories of borderline patients and significantly more common among their childhood histories than among the childhood histories of other diagnostic groups (Akiskal, Chen, et al. 1985; Bradley, 1979; Links, Steiner, Offord, & Eppel, 1988; Paris, Zweig-Frank, & Guzder, 1994a; Soloff & Millward 1983; Walsh, 1977; Zanarini, Gunderson, Marino, Schwartz, & Frankenburg, 1989; Zanarini et al.,

1997). Only one study found that these experiences were not discriminating for BPD (Paris, Zweig-Frank, & Guzder, 1994b).

Studies of Disturbed Parental Involvement

Three conclusions have emerged from these studies (Frank & Hoffman, 1986; Frank & Paris, 1981; Goldberg, Mann, Wise, & Segall, 1985; Grinker, Werble, & Drye, 1968; Gunderson, Kerr, & Englund, 1986; Paris & Frank, 1989; Soloff & Millward, 1983; Walsh, 1977). The first is that patients with BPD usually see their relationships with their mothers as highly conflictual, distant, or uninvolved. The second is that the failure of fathers to be present and involved is an even more discriminating aspect of these families than a problematic relationship with their mother. The third is that disturbed relationships with both parents may be both more specific for BPD and pathogenic than that with either parent alone.

Studies of Childhood Verbal and Emotional Abuse

Two studies have assessed the prevalence of these forms of abuse in the childhood histories of borderline patients and comparison subjects (Zanarini, Gunderson, Marino, et al., 1989; Zanarini et al., 1997). Two main findings have emerged from these studies. First, these experiences are extremely common among borderline patients. Second, they are significantly more common among the reported childhood experiences of borderline patients than among the reported childhood experiences of depressed and Axis II comparison subjects.

Studies of Childhood Physical and Sexual Abuse

Ten studies have assessed the childhood histories of physical and/or sexual abuse reported by borderline adolescents or adults (Herman, Perry,

& van der Kolk, 1989; Links, Steiner, Offord, et al., 1988; Ogata et al., 1990; Paris et al., 1994a; Paris et al., 1994b; Salzman et al., 1993; Shearer, Peters, Quaytman, & Ogden, 1990; Westen, Ludolph, Misle, Ruffins, & Block, 1990; Zanarini, Gunderson, Marino, et al., 1989; Zanarini et al., 1997). Four main findings have emerged from these studies. First, both physical and sexual abuse are relatively common in the childhood histories of criteria-defined borderline patients. Second, physical abuse is generally not reported significantly more often by borderline patients than by comparison subjects. Third, sexual abuse is consistently reported significantly more often by borderline patients than depressed or personality-disordered comparison subjects. Fourth, borderline patients with milder cases of BPD report lower rates of childhood sexual abuse than those with more severe cases of BPD (e.g., Salzman et al., 1993, vs. Zanarini et al., 1997). They also tend to report less severe forms of abuse (e.g., mostly one-time abuse [Paris et al., 1994a and 1994b] vs. mostly ongoing abuse [Zanarini et al., 1997]).

Studies of Childhood Physical and Emotional Neglect

Four studies have assessed one or more forms of reported childhood neglect in borderline patients and comparison subjects (Ogata et al., 1990; Westen et al., 1990; Zanarini, Gunderson, Marino, et al. 1989; Zanarini et al., 1997). Three main findings have emerged from these studies. First, physical neglect, which is relatively uncommon among borderline patients, was only found to be significantly more common among borderline patients in two of these studies (Westen et al., 1990; Zanarini et al., 1997). Second, emotional neglect is very common among borderline patients and highly discriminating for the disorder. Third, emotional neglect is multifaceted and each of the constituent facets studied (emotional withdrawal, inconsistent treatment, denial of feelings, lack of a real relationship, parentification of patient, and failure to provide needed protection) is significantly more common among borderline patients than among comparison subjects (Zanarini et al., 1997).

STATE OF CURRENT KNOWLEDGE CONCERNING
CHILDHOOD ADVERSITY

The existing empirical evidence strongly suggests that a high percentage of borderline patients report unfortunate or traumatic experiences occurring during their childhood. These studies also suggest that most forms of childhood adversity are reported by a significantly higher percentage of borderline patients than comparison subjects. In addition, studies have found that many of these forms of adversity co-occur (Zanarini et al., 1997; Zanarini, Frankenburg, et al., 2000).

In general, both patients and clinicians treating them tend to view experiences of frank abuse or neglect as being more serious than experiences of early separations and loss, or disturbed parental involvement. But are they? And if so, how much more serious? Is the death of a parent when the potentially borderline child is two or three years of age 10% or 30% less serious than being sexually abused by an adult neighbor at the age of 11 or 12? Or given the young age of the child, is the death 20% or 60% more serious?

It is our belief that these types of comparisons are not useful, and each patient's history must be examined on its own to determine its effect on that particular patient's borderline psychopathology. After all, pain is not a competitive sport, and heartbreak is not an easily quantifiable commodity. But more importantly, different patients may have had similar experiences of adversity but may believe, with good reason, that different types of adversity were the most painful part of their childhood.

SYNTHESIS OF THE ETIOLOGY OF THE INNER PAIN
OF BORDERLINE PATIENTS

Clinical experience suggests that some or much of the pain of being borderline is related to adverse childhood events or experiences. Clinical experience also suggests that some of the pain of being borderline comes from their inborn temperament. Studies have found that BPD is associated with a temperament characterized by a high degree of neuroticism (i.e., emotional pain) as well as a low degree of agreeableness (i.e., strong individuality) (Clarkin, Hull, Cantor, & Sanderson, 1993; Morey & Zanarini, 2000; Trull, Widiger, Lynam, & Costa, 2003; Wilberg, Urnes, Friis, Pederson, & Karterud, 1999). In addition, twin studies have found that these two aspects of normal personality as measured by the Five Factor Model are highly heritable (Jang, Livesley, & Vernon, 1996; Jang, McCrae, Angleitner, Reimann, & Livesley, 1998).

It is also likely that these factors—childhood adversity and a vulnerable temperament—interact with one another in ways that are not useful. For example, a youngster with a highly sensitive and hypervigilant nature may be particularly affected by inconsistent parental treatment. But his objections only further upset his parents, who then may emotionally withdraw from him, verbally attack him, or both.

Kindling Events or Experiences of a Normative Nature

We had previously mentioned kindling events of a normative nature. These experiences tend to occur outside of the family and typically require that a child, adolescent, or young adult is trying to act in an increasingly autonomous and competent manner. Attending school, having friends, and dating are three of the most common and developmentally important areas. But some potentially borderline persons cannot function very well on their own, having problems with autonomy, competence, or some admixture of the two. Clinical experience suggests that there are two responses to this type of perceived failure. One is to turn to one's parents for help. In some cases, they are able to provide the guidance and support that the potentially borderline person needs. But in some cases, they are not. More common is the situation where the potential BPD patient develops a "theory" of the problem that holds her parents responsible for her failures, which might involve having trouble completing schoolwork, having few friends, or rarely dating. Her parents, in turn, resent being blamed for what they see as a personal defeat, and intense intrafamilial fighting ensues. This fighting can reach such a level of intensity that the never-treated young person is suddenly hospitalized on an emergency basis and officially becomes the "identified" patient.

ETIOLOGY OF THE BEHAVIORAL AND INTERPERSONAL STRATEGIES CHARACTERISTIC OF BPD

Why do so many borderline patients engage in self-mutilation, one of the most discriminating symptoms of BPD (Zanarini, Gunderson, Frankenburg, & Chauncey, 1990)? Why do so many make help-seeking suicide threats and gestures, another of the most discriminating symptoms of BPD (Zanarini, Gunderson, Frankenburg, & Chauncey 1990)? Why do borderline patients behave in such a troubling and troublesome manner when interacting with people upon whom they depend? Why do they manipulate people rather than asking for help in a direct manner? Why do they devalue other people and their strengths and achievements? Why do they act as if they are entitled to special treatment? Why are they so demanding?

It would be easy to blame their impulsive patterns and interpersonal behavior on their biology. Many observers believe that BPD is the outward manifestation of the psychobiological dimensions first described by Siever and Davis (1991), particularly affective lability and impulsivity. And yet, many people suffer from problems with mood lability and impulsivity but do not meet criteria for BPD. In addition, and perhaps more germane to the discussion at hand, many labile, impulsive people do not arouse the negative feelings that many borderline patients do.

Six of the seven studies that have assessed the familial risk of developing BPD have found that BPD "breeds true": that is, it is significantly more common among the first-degree relatives of borderline patients than among the first-degree relatives of schizophrenic, depressed, bipolar, Axis II, or normal comparison subjects (Baron, Gruen, Asnis, & Lord,

1985; Gunderson, Zanarini et al., 2011; Links, Steiner, & Huxley, 1988; Loranger, Oldham, & Tulis, 1982; Zanarini, Gunderson, Marino, Schwartz, & Frankenburg, 1988; Zanarini, Frankenburg, Yong, et al., 2004). Studies that have assessed the familial prevalence of the symptoms of BPD have found that they are more common in the first-degree relatives of borderline patients than BPD itself (Gunderson, Zanarini et al., 2011; Silverman et al., 1991; Zanarini, Frankenburg, Yong, et al., 2004). They have also found that these symptoms are significantly more common among the first-degree relatives of borderline patients than the first-degree relatives of comparison subjects.

Does this mean that people inherit these symptoms, learn about them through family interactions, or some combination of the two? Given the nature of these studies, there is currently no clear answer to these questions. However, the results of three large-scale twin studies suggest that BPD itself is highly heritable (Reichborn-Kjennerud et al., 2013; Torgersen et al., 2000; Torgerson et al., 2012). Studies of BPD in the community have also found it be heritable (Gunderson, Zanarini, et al., 2011; Kendler, Myers, & Reichborn-Kjennerud, 2011).

Based on clinical experience, we believe that these impulsive and interpersonal behaviors once worked to help manage the pain of being borderline. Perhaps more accurately, these maneuvers may have contributed to such turmoil in the family that the child or adolescent was temporarily distracted from his or her pain. The resulting interpersonal struggles were usually so action-packed that there was little time to feel much of anything. Unfortunately, these struggles also served to affirm the deeply held but mistaken belief that other people are uncaring or malevolent.

This pattern of struggling with others to avoid experiencing inner pain may have been tolerated in the family. However, it is more difficult to get friends and romantic partners to tolerate such behavior for extended periods of time. This is also true of borderline patients' dealings with many mental health professionals. Ultimately, this type of collaborative turmoil has seriously interfered with the child or adolescent learning to handle his or her distress in a more straightforward, adaptive manner.

In fact, many borderline patients are unaware that their behavior is causing more problems than it is solving. They know that something about them is off-putting, but they may not be able to correctly identify what that something is. They may, for example, believe that they are not getting the help they need because other people are repelled by their imperfections. However, the more parsimonious explanation may be that people do not like being accused of being mean or uncaring.

Borderline psychopathology has long been thought to fall into four symptom sectors: affective symptoms, cognitive symptoms, behavioral or impulsive symptoms, and interpersonal symptoms. This complex theory of borderline psychopathology provides a model that describes the role of all four sectors of this psychopathology. Pain of either an affective and/or cognitive nature is first aroused, and then behavioral and/or interpersonal symptoms are brought to bear to help manage this pain. More specifically, they help to hide its depth from both the patient and those who become involved in trying to help him manage his impulsivity and his often turbulent relationships.

However, it is possible that the cascade of symptoms can begin in any sector and then spread out to the others. It may be different for different patients or for the same patient at different times.

Before beginning to focus on the findings of the McLean Study of Adult Development, or MSAD, we will review the findings of 21 earlier studies of the course of BPD: 17 small-scale studies of the short-term course of BPD, and four large-scale, follow-back studies of the long-term course of BPD.

3

Earlier Studies of the Longitudinal Course of BPD

Before the McLean Study of Adult Development (MSAD) began, or during its first years of data collection, our knowledge about the course of BPD was based on 17 small-scale, short-term, prospective studies and four large-scale, long-term, follow-back studies of the course and outcome of BPD. This chapter will review the results of both of these types of studies.

SMALL-SCALE, SHORT-TERM, PROSPECTIVE STUDIES OF THE COURSE OF BPD

In this section, we first review three distinct groups of short-term studies that were conducted in the 1960s–1970s, 1980s, and 1990s.

The Early Studies: 1960s–1970s

The early studies assessed the social functioning, employment status, and rehospitalization rates of very small numbers (14–41) of people

hospitalized with what we would today call "borderline personality disorder." As prospective studies, they identified a group of individuals with
borderline symptoms or a diagnosis of BPD, and followed them forward
through time to monitor their course and outcome. (There may or may not
have been a comparison group of individuals with a different treatment or
disorder in any given study.) The advantages of prospective studies are
that they begin with "baseline" observations and are not as affected by re-
call bias as retrospective studies.

In the first of these early studies, Grinker and associates (1968)
followed 41 patients at a mean of 2.5 years after hospitalization and
found that two-thirds of the patients described themselves as worse
off, the same, or only marginally improved since their index hospitalization. Although one-third required rehospitalization during the
follow-up period, the majority were occupationally stable but working
in low-level jobs. Their social functioning was comparatively more impaired, with most having limited leisure-time activities and transient
contact with people. Nearly half of the patients had troubled or min-
imal relationships with their families.

Werble (1970) published a six- to seven-year follow-up of 28 of the same
patients and found that most lived in the community; about half had been
rehospitalized, but only briefly. They continued to work, but were socially
isolated, having little contact with either family or friends.

Gunderson and his colleagues studied the two-year course of a group
of 24 patients given a borderline diagnosis, matched by age, sex, race, and
socioeconomic status with 29 patients with schizophrenia (Gunderson,
Carpenter, & Strauss, 1975). They found that, on average, these patients
had been employed part-time to full-time for much of the year prior to
follow-up, had social contacts about every other week, and had been
hospitalized for less than three months during the previous year. Their
signs and symptoms were described as both moderate and intermittent.
In every area, the borderline patients remained as functionally impaired
as the schizophrenic comparison group.

Carpenter and Gunderson (1977) followed 14 of the original 24
patients five years after their initial diagnosis. Their functioning was still

indistinguishable from that of the schizophrenic group, except that the borderline patients maintained the quality of their social contacts, while those of the schizophrenic patients deteriorated. Relatively few had required hospitalization. Although several were "loners," most met regularly with friends. Almost all patients were employed continuously, although some were under-employed. Overall, their functioning had not changed significantly since their two-year follow-up.

Studies Conducted in the 1980s

This group of studies reflects the use of the operationalized *Diagnostic and Statistical Manual of Mental Disorders, 3rd ed. (DSM-III)* criteria for BPD, which were introduced, as noted before, into our nomenclature in 1980. These studies examine the occurrence of comorbid (or coexisting) disorders, including alcohol and drug abuse, rates of rehospitalization, and occupational and social functioning.

Pope and associates applied the new criteria retrospectively to a group of patients by reviewing their medical records (Pope, Jonas, Hudson, Cohen, & Gunderson, 1983). They followed 27 of 33 patients with BPD as defined by *DSM-III* for four to seven years after their index hospitalization. Two-thirds of these patients had a probable or definite diagnosis of BPD at follow-up. As a whole, the group of patients with BPD had a significantly worse outcome than comparison groups with bipolar or schizoaffective disorders. They were similar to a comparison group with schizophrenia on most outcome indices, except that the BPD patients had significantly better occupational functioning.

Pope and colleagues (1983) were also the first to study comorbid diagnoses of borderline patients and their effect on outcome. They compared patients with "pure" BPD with those having a concurrent major affective (or mood) disorder, and found that the BPD patients with an affective disorder were functioning better socially and had fewer symptoms. The researchers linked this finding to the fact that these patients were more likely to have had a positive response to medication.

Akiskal and coworkers (1985) also studied the occurrence of mood disorders in BPD, and found that half of the 100 outpatients with BPD they followed over a period of six months to three years developed a mood disorder during the follow-up period. These disorders included major depression, manic episodes, hypomanic episodes, and mixed affective disorders. Many of these patients had a diagnosis of concurrent mood disorder at the beginning of the study, but even in the group that had no initial diagnosis of affective disorder, 11 patients had an episode of major depression, and four committed suicide. These investigators hypothesized that borderline personality might represent an atypical form of bipolar disorder.

Also in 1985, Barasch and colleagues conducted a three-year follow-up of 10 patients with *DSM-III* diagnosed BPD and a reference group of 20 patients with other *DSM-III* personality disorders (Barasch, Frances, Hurt, Clarkin, & Cohen, 1985). They found that the two groups were similar in their functioning and the slight degree of their improvement over the follow-up period. Forty percent of each group developed a major depressive episode during the follow-up period. Thus, neither the degree of their impairment nor their level of affective symptomatology distinguished the two groups. In addition, these researchers assessed the degree of stability of the borderline diagnosis over the follow-up period. Sixty percent of the BPD group met *DSM-III* criteria for BPD at follow-up, and 30% met four (rather than the required five) *DSM-III* criteria. Of the 20 non-borderline subjects, only three met *DSM-III* BPD criteria at follow-up. The authors concluded that BPD was a stable diagnosis over time and that it was neither a variant of major depression nor a nonspecific label for severe personality disorders.

Perry and Cooper (1985) compared a group of 30 borderline patients with a group of patients diagnosed with *DSM-III* antisocial personality disorder (APD) and a group of patients with bipolar II disorder one to three years after their initial assessment. They used a semi-structured diagnostic interview to assess the presence of *DSM-III* BPD. With regard to global functioning, these investigators found that the mean Global Assessment Score (GAS) (Endicott, Spitzer, Fleiss, & Cohen, 1976) for their BPD group was 51 at baseline, which is considered to be in the "fair" range. They also found no differences on this measure among their three groups at two- to three-year follow-up. However, a continuous measure of borderline pathology was predictive of both lower GAS scores and greater variability in functioning. During the follow-up period, Perry and Cooper (1985) found several differences between BPD and APD patients. They found that the patients with BPD used significantly more psychiatric services (after controlling for gender), and that borderline patients without antisocial pathology were more depressed and anxious.

Nace, Saxon, and Shore (1986) studied 59 alcoholic inpatients diagnosed with the criteria of the original Diagnostic Interview for Borderlines (DIB) (Gunderson, Kolb, & Austin, 1981). Thirteen met criteria for BPD and were found to have a significant decrease in their use of alcohol at one-year follow-up, a significant improvement in satisfaction with their home and family situation as well as their use of leisure time, and a significant decrease in their number of hospitalizations. When compared to non-borderline alcoholics, those with BPD were significantly more likely to be using drugs (but not alcohol) during the follow-up year. They were also significantly more likely to be working and significantly less likely to have a good relationship with their parents.

Tucker and colleagues studied 40 patients with "borderline disorders"— not necessarily *DSM-III* BPD—who were hospitalized on a specialized long-term treatment unit (Tucker, Bauer, Wagner, Harlam, & Sher, 1987). Two years after discharge, these patients had less suicidal ideation and behavior, were more likely to be in continuous psychotherapy, and had more close friendships and positive relationships than at baseline. Those hospitalized for more than 12 months were less likely to be rehospitalized and more likely to be in continuous psychotherapy during the first year following discharge, but these differences disappeared after the first year. The mean GAS score for this sample was 29.7 at admission, 41.6 at discharge, 50.3 one year after discharge, and 56.5 two years after discharge, indicating that these patients moved from the "incapacitated" to the "fair" range of functioning over time.

In 1989, Modestin and Villiger compared Swiss patients with BPD to Swiss patients with other personality disorders. After following 18 *DSM-III* diagnosed borderline patients and 17 personality-disordered patients with heterogeneous non-borderline diagnoses for 4.5 years, they found that BPD patients were quite impaired, with about 70% only working part-time or receiving a disability pension. However, these patients functioned at about the same vocational and social level as the comparison group, with the exception that significantly fewer were married. These investigators also found that BPD patients were more often rehospitalized, but their hospitalizations were of shorter duration. However, both groups exhibited the same high level of depressive and anxiety symptoms.

Small Studies During the 1990s

These studies originated mainly from Canada and Northern Europe and focused on social and occupational functioning, the stability of the diagnosis of BPD over time, and also on the parameters of various psychiatric treatments. Links and his associates studied 88 Canadian inpatients diagnosed with BPD by the DIB and found that 40% of the 65 subjects who were re-interviewed two years after their index admission no longer met these criteria (Links, Mitton, & Steiner, 1990). They also found that 20% of their borderline subjects were employed full-time for the entire follow-up period, 83% had weekly contact with friends, 60% were hospitalized for less than 5% of the follow-up period, and 69% were in continuous outpatient treatment for about a year. At the time of the second follow-up (Links, Heslegrave, Mitton, Van Reekum, & Patrick, 1995; Links, Heslegrave, & Van Reekum, 1998), these investigators found that patients in the study group who were symptomatic were significantly more likely than those in remission (53%) to have major depression, dysthymia, and other Axis II disorders, particularly, anxious cluster personality disorders. They also had significantly more episodes of substance abuse/dependence than those in remission, and were more dependent on disability payments than those in remission.

Mehlum and colleagues (1991) studied 34 day-hospital patients in Norway who received a clinical diagnosis of BPD. When 25 of these patients were reassessed two to five years later, their overall Health Sickness Rating Scale (HSRS; Luborsky, 1962) score rose from a mean of 39 to a mean of 49—a significant improvement, but still in the marginal range of functioning. More than half were employed, 39% were self-supporting, and 48% had been hospitalized (for a mean of 11% of the follow-up period). Additionally, these 25 patients had spent 41% of the time they were followed in therapy and 32% of the time on medication.

In an Australian study, Stevenson and Meares (1992) followed 30 outpatients enrolled in an intensive course of standardized psychotherapy. All 30 met *DSM-III* criteria for BPD at baseline, but 30% had experienced a remission by the time the 12-month treatment program had ended.

Linehan, Heard, et al. (1993) studied 39 women with DIB-diagnosed BPD one year after they finished a year of randomized treatment with either dialectical behavioral therapy (DBT) or treatment as usual. The DBT group had significantly fewer episodes of parasuicidal behavior at 18 months (but not 24 months) than those in the comparison group.

In addition to social functioning, the next two studies examined the use of medications in the groups of patients followed. Sandell and associates (1993) studied 132 broadly defined borderline patients in day treatment in Sweden. They followed 86 patients 3–10 years later through a mailed questionnaire and found that 26% were engaged in full-time work, 34% were on disability, 26% were married or living together, and 47% were living alone. They also found that 12% had been prescribed anxiolytics, 29% antipsychotics, and 6% antidepressants.

Antikainen and coworkers studied 62 broadly defined borderline patients who had been treated on a long-term inpatient unit in Finland designed specifically for patients with BPD (Antikainen, Hintikka, Lehtonen, Koponen, & Arstila, 1995). Forty-two patients participated in the follow-up interview three years later. Sixty-four percent had been unable to work for at least one year, and 33% were currently married. Forty-five percent had been hospitalized, 52% were in therapy, 67% had been prescribed anxiolytics, 40% antipsychotics, and 52% antidepressants.

Najavits and Gunderson (1995) followed 37 female inpatients diagnosed with the DIB who were beginning a new psychotherapy. Thirty-three were re-interviewed one year after their entry into the study, 23 two years after this, and 20 three years after their first assessment. Their GAS score increased from 44 at baseline to 57 three years later, indicating that, as a group, the remaining subjects moved from the "marginal" to the "fair" range of functioning.

Senol and colleagues studied 61 clinically diagnosed borderline inpatients in Turkey, 45 of whom consented to a follow-up interview two to four years after their index admission (Senol, Dereboy, & Yuksel, 1997). Their mean GAS score increased from 41 to 46, a statistically significant but clinically minor difference. It was also found that only 4% experienced a remission of their BPD, but that 54% had met criteria for a mood disorder, and 56% had met criteria for a substance use disorder during the follow-up period.

LESSONS LEARNED FROM SHORT-TERM STUDIES

The results of these short-term, prospective studies have generally been interpreted to mean that most borderline patients were doing relatively poorly one to seven years after their initial evaluation. While all of these studies of the course of BPD provided useful information, and many were considered state of the art at the time that they were conducted, all of them suffered from one or more methodological problems that limited what could be generalized from their results. Chief among these limitations were the following: small sample sizes, high attrition rates, the absence of comparison groups or the use of psychotic comparison groups, lack of explicit criteria for BPD, the use of unstructured assessment techniques for making diagnoses, non-blinded assessment of outcome status, limited assessment of outcome functioning, varying length of follow-up within the same study, and only one follow-up wave for most of these studies.

Despite these limitations, three major findings concerning the short-term course of BPD have emerged from these studies. First, borderline patients continued to have substantial difficulty functioning six months to seven years after their initial assessment, particularly in the areas of social functioning. Second, a substantial percentage continued to need psychiatric care, particularly outpatient treatment. Third, their borderline psychopathology was reasonably stable, with five (out of 17 studies) reporting rates of remission between 4% and 53%, with a median value of 32%.

LARGE-SCALE, LONG-TERM, FOLLOW-BACK STUDIES OF THE COURSE OF BPD

Follow-back studies have the advantage of using treatment records to locate large numbers of patients with a particular diagnosis. However, a major disadvantage is that researchers have to use the variable information found in medical records to make study diagnoses. In the first of these large-scale studies, Plakun and associates conducted a follow-back study of 237 patients who had been hospitalized between 1950 and 1976 at Austen Riggs, a private psychiatric hospital in western Massachusetts (Plakun, Burkhardt, & Muller, 1985). They had originally mailed out a 50-item questionnaire to the 878 patients who had been hospitalized for at least two months, and they received a 27% response rate (another potential drawback to this type of study). Among those diagnosed through chart review according to *DSM-III* criteria were the following patient groups: 61 borderline patients, 19 schizophrenic patients, 24 patients with major affective disorder, 13 schizotypal patients, and 19 patients with schizoid personality disorder. At a mean follow-up period of 15 years, the borderline patients achieved a mean GAS of 67, a score in the "good" range of functioning. Both the 54 "aggregated" borderlines (all but those with a coexisting major mood disorder) and the borderline patients with a comorbid schizotypal disorder achieved a higher mean GAS than the schizophrenic patients. In addition, borderline patients without a comorbid affective disorder were functioning significantly better than those who also had a mood disorder.

In the second large-scale study, McGlashan (1986) followed up all inpatients treated at Chestnut Lodge between 1950 and 1975 who met the following criteria: (1) index admission of at least 90 days; (2) age between 16 and 55; and (3) absence of an organic brain syndrome. Follow-up information was obtained on 446 patients, resulting in a trace rate of 72%, and was collected by the use of a semi-structured clinical interview by telephone with the patient or an informant. Most comparisons focused on 81 patients only meeting criteria for BPD, 163 who met criteria for schizophrenia, and 44 who met criteria for major depression, with diagnoses being derived through retrospective chart review.

McGlashan (1986) found that his borderline patients achieved an overall HSRS score of 64 a mean of 15 years after their index admission (range 2–32 years). This mean rating represents a good level of functioning and was equal to that of depressed comparison subjects, but significantly higher than that of schizophrenic patients. However, closer examination reveals that although half of the borderline patients (53%) were functioning in the good–recovered range, the other half (47%) were functioning in the moderate–incapacitated range. In addition, 3% of the traced borderline patients had committed suicide. In terms of instrumental functioning, those with BPD worked about half the time at reasonably complex jobs. They also met with friends about once every other week. About half were married or living with a sexual partner, and about half avoided intimate relationships entirely. In terms of further treatment, the average borderline patient was rehospitalized one or two more times, spending about 8% of the follow-up period as an inpatient. They used psychosocial treatments during about one-third of the follow-up period (35%) and psychotropic medications about one-fourth of the time (22%). Almost half (46%) were in some form of psychiatric treatment at the time of their follow-up interview. These figures were very similar to those achieved by the depressed controls. However, the borderline patients functioned significantly better than schizophrenic patients in the instrumental realm and used significantly less psychiatric treatment than these psychotic comparison subjects.

McGlashan (1986) found that overall functioning was significantly related to the length of the follow-up period. He found that patients who were followed for 10–19 years had significantly better overall functioning than those followed nine years or less and about the same level of functioning as those followed 20 years or more. He also found that overall functioning of these patients over time followed the pattern of an inverted U, with functioning improving through their 20s and 30s, peaking in their 40s, and declining in their 50s.

In the third study, Paris and colleagues reviewed the charts of all patients hospitalized for psychiatric reasons at the Jewish General Hospital in Montreal between 1958 and 1978 (Paris, Brown, & Nowlis, 1987). Three hundred twenty-two patients met retrospective DIB criteria for BPD, and 100 of these patients (32%) were re-interviewed a mean of 15 years after their first admission. The researchers found that all aspects of their borderline psychopathology as measured by a DIB interview had decreased significantly. They also found that only 25% of these patients still met DIB criteria for BPD. In terms of overall functioning, these borderline patients achieved a mean HSRS score of 63, a score indicating a good global outcome. They also achieved a mean work score of 3.8, indicating frequent job changes without unemployment. Their social participation score was 3.2, close to a level described as limited leisure time with transient social contact. In terms of further treatment, they had a mean of 1.3 rehospitalizations and a mean of 1.9 years of further treatment. Overall, there was great variability in the amount of treatment received, but most of the patients' treatment histories were chaotic and intermittent. Of the165 patients who could be located, 14 (9%) had committed suicide.

Paris and Zweig-Frank (2001) later reassessed this sample of borderline patients a mean of 27 years after their first admission. They found that only five of the 64 (8%) once-borderline inpatients interviewed met the more restrictive Revised Diagnostic Interview for Borderlines (DIB-R) criteria for BPD (Zanarini, Gunderson, Frankenburg, & Chauncey, 1989). Additionally, 83% had been married or lived with a partner at some point, and 59% had children. However, their mean Global Assessment of Functioning (GAF) score still had not progressed to the "recovered" range, and 10% of the original borderline cohort had committed suicide by the time of their second follow-up assessment.

In the last of these large-scale studies, Stone (1990) followed up 502 (91%) of the 550 patients hospitalized at the New York State Psychiatric Institute between 1963 and 1976 meeting the following inclusion criteria: (1) a stay of at least three months; (2) age under 40; and (3) an IQ of 90 or higher. Most of these patients had originally been selected for admission to the hospital for their potential to benefit from intensive psychotherapy. However, a substantial minority were admitted because of their family's VIP status. Stone made retrospective *DSM-III* diagnoses after reviewing each patient's chart and then attempted to contact each patient personally, most of whom he had known during their index hospitalization. He was able to trace 193 (94%) of the 206 patients meeting *DSM-III* criteria for BPD and interviewed relatives or other informants when patients were unavailable. Stone found that the average GAS score of this group of patients a mean of 16 years after their index admission was 67. This score, which indicates a good level of functioning, was significantly higher than that achieved by schizophrenic comparison subjects. Almost half of the surviving borderline patients received a GAS score in the recovered range (41%), 28% received a GAS score in the good range, 18% in the fair range, and 13% in the marginal-incapacitated range. This distribution was also significantly different from that attained by the schizophrenic patients in the study, with only 6% of these patients receiving GAS scores in the recovered range.

In terms of more specific spheres of follow-up functioning, 53% of the borderline patients had worked at least three-quarters of the time, 17% had worked about half the time, and 30% worked less than half the time or not at all. Less than half (45%) had ever married, and less than a quarter (23%) had children. However, only 28% had ever been rehospitalized or spent time in another institution. In addition, borderline patients functioned better in each of these spheres than schizophrenic patients. Despite these generally optimistic findings, it is important to note that 9% percent of these *DSM-III* borderlines committed suicide, a rate identical to that found for schizophrenic patients, but substantially lower than that found for patients with schizoaffective disorder (23%).

LESSONS LEARNED FROM THE FOLLOW-BACK
STUDIES

In contrast to the short-term prospective studies described earlier in the chapter, the results of these long-term, follow-back studies have generally been interpreted to mean that most borderline patients were doing reasonably well a mean of 14–16 years after their index admission. Despite the consistency of the findings in these four studies, the generalizability of their results is limited by a number of methodological problems that also hindered the generalizability of the short-term studies described earlier in the chapter. These problems have included: the use of highly variable chart material as the basis for diagnoses; assessment of post-hospital functioning at only one point in time in three of the four studies; absence of detailed information concerning follow-up functioning; lack of independence of baseline and follow-up data; absence of comparison subjects or failure to use near-neighbor Axis II comparison subjects. More specific to these long-term studies were: the use of mailed questionnaires or telephone interviews as the only or primary source of information; interviewing of relatives or other informants in some cases; use of upper-middle-class inpatient samples from tertiary facilities in three of the four studies; the wide range of follow-up periods in each of these studies; and the presence of different age cohorts.

Despite these limitations, one major finding has emerged from these studies: the functioning of borderline patients over time is highly variable, with some functioning very well, many continuing to have substantial difficulty in a number of areas of their lives, and 3–10% committing suicide. In addition, only one study assessed remission rates, and this study found rates of 75% at a mean of 15 years and 92% at a mean of 27 years.

Recognizing the gap in our knowledge resulting from these methodologically less-than-optimal short and long-term studies of the course of BPD, the National Institute of Mental Health (NIMH) funded the MSAD study, which will be the focus of the rest of this book. They also funded the Collaborative Longitudinal Personality Disorders Study (CLPS) four years later (Gunderson, Stout, et al., 2011). This methodologically rigorous study, on which I was a co-investigator, followed subjects with BPD, schizotypal personality disorder, avoidant personality disorder, obsessive compulsive personality disorder, and major depression without serious personality psychopathology for a decade. It differed from MSAD in following five rather than two study groups. It also differed in that these groups were not mutually exclusive. And for the most part, they were reassessed every year rather than every two years.

4

The McLean Study of Adult Development (MSAD)

RESEARCH DESIGN AND MEASURES

All patients in the McLean Study of Adult Development (MSAD) were between the ages of 18 and 35, had an IQ of 71 or higher, and were fluent in English. In addition, none had ever met criteria for schizophrenia, schizoaffective disorder, bipolar I disorder, or been diagnosed with a serious organic condition that could cause serious psychiatric symptoms (e.g., multiple sclerosis, systemic lupus erythematosus).

After signing an informed consent form, each patient met with our research team three times during his or her index admission, which averaged six days in length. The first meeting concerned premorbid psychosocial functioning, previous psychiatric treatment, borderline psychopathology, and co-occurring Axis I and II disorders. At this meeting, five semi-structured interviews were administered: the Baseline Information Schedule (BIS) (Zanarini, Frankenburg, Khera, & Bleichmar, 2001), the Structured Clinical Interview for *DSM-III-R* Axis I Disorders (SCID

I) (Spitzer, Williams, Gibbon, & First, 1992), the Revised Diagnostic
Interview for Borderlines (DIB-R) (Zanarini, Gunderson, Frankenburg,
et al., 1989), the Lifetime Self-Destructiveness Scale (LSDS) (Zanarini,
Frankenburg, Reich, et al., 2008), and the Revised Diagnostic Interview
for *DSM-III-R* Personality Disorders (DIPD-R) (Zanarini, Frankenburg,
Chauncey, & Gunderson, 1987).

The second meeting, which was conducted blind to the patient's diagnostic status, concerned family history of psychiatric disorder, psychiatric disorders in environmentally important others (e.g., step-parents,
spouses), and pathological and protective childhood experiences. At this
meeting, three other semi-structured interviews were administered: the
Revised Family History Questionnaire (FHQ-R) (Zanarini, et al.,
1988), the Revised Childhood Experiences Questionnaire (CEQ-R)
(Zanarini, Gunderson, Frankenburg, et al., 1989), and the Abuse History
Interview (AHI) (Zanarini, Frankenburg, Marino, Reich, Haynes, &
Gunderson, 1999).

At a third meeting, each patient filled out five self-report instruments.
These measures were: the Dissociative Experiences Scale (DES)
(Bernstein & Putnam, 1986), the Dysphoric Affect Scale (DAS) (Zanarini,
Frankenburg, DeLuca, 1998), the Positive Affect Scale (PAS) (Reed &
Zanarini, 2011), the Five-Factor NEO Inventory of Personality (NEO-
FFI) (Costa & McCrae, 1992), and the Defense Style Questionnaire (DSQ)
(Bond, 1992).

At each follow-up wave, each patient was first sent a letter indicating that
his or her follow-up date was approaching. Each patient was then contacted
by phone, and a mutually convenient time and place for the follow-up interview was arranged. At this interview, which covered the preceding two
years, informed consent was obtained. Then six semi-structured interviews
were administered: the Revised Borderline Follow-up Interview (BFI-R)
(the follow-up analog to the BIS) (Zanarini, Frankenburg, Hennen, et al.,
2005), a change version of the SCID I (covering only the preceding two
years), the DIB-R, the follow-up version of the LSDS, the DIPD-R, and
the follow-up version of the AHI. Five self-report instruments were also

re-administered at this time: the DES, the DAS, the PAS, the NEO-FFI, and the DSQ. Each follow-up evaluation was conducted blind to baseline diagnosis by an interviewer with at least two years of clinical experience working with personality-disordered patients.

With the six-year wave, we added two semi-structured interviews to our assessment battery, and these have been re-administered at each subsequent wave: the Life Events Assessment (LEA) (Shrout, et al., 1989) and the Medical History and Services Utilization Interview (MHSUI) (Frankenburg & Zanarini, 2004a). We also added a (one time only) measure to assess intelligence (the Shipley Institute of Living Scale [Zachary, 1994]).

SUBJECTS

All told, the baseline diagnostic interviews were administered to 378 consecutive inpatients at McLean Hospital who were thought to meet inclusion/exclusion criteria. Two hundred and ninety patients met both DIB-R and *DSM-III-R* criteria for BPD, and 72 met *DSM-III-R* criteria for at least one non-borderline Axis II disorder (and neither criteria set for BPD). Sixteen others were excluded from further study because they either met criteria for schizophrenia (N = 2) or bipolar I disorder (N = 2) or failed to meet *DSM-III-R* criteria for any Axis II disorder (N = 12).

Of the 72 comparison subjects, 4% met *DSM-III-R* criteria for an odd cluster personality disorder, 33% met *DSM-III-R* criteria for an anxious cluster personality disorder, and 18% met *DSM-III-R* criteria for a non-borderline dramatic cluster personality disorder. An additional 53% met *DSM-III-R* criteria for personality disorder not otherwise specified (PDNOS) (which was operationally defined in the DIPD-R as meeting all but one of the required number of criteria for at least two of the 13 Axis II disorders described in *DSM-III-R*).

At baseline, borderline patients and Axis II comparison subjects were very similar in terms of mean age (about 27) and racial background (less

than 15% nonwhite). However, a significantly higher percentage of borderline patients than Axis II comparison subjects were female (80.3% vs.
63.9%). In addition, borderline patients came from a significantly lower
mean socioeconomic background (3.4 vs. 2.8) as measured by the five-
point Hollingshead-Redlich scale (1 = highest, 5 = lowest) (Hollingshead,
1957) and had a significantly lower mean GAF score than Axis II comparison subjects (38.9 vs. 43.5) (although both groups had a mean GAF score
in the impaired range).

SAMPLE RETENTION

MSAD began 26 years ago. We completed eight waves of blind follow-up
a number of years ago: two, four, six, eight, 10, 12, 14, and 16-year follow-
up evaluations. In addition, we just recently completed the 18- and 20-
year follow-up waves. The 22-year and 24-year waves of follow-up will be
completed in about a year.

The trace rate in this series of patients has remained extremely high
over time. In terms of continuing participation, 87.5% (N = 231/264) of
surviving borderline patients (13 died by suicide and 13 died of other
causes) were re-interviewed at all eight follow-up waves that have been
completed. A similar rate of participation was found for Axis II comparison subjects, with 82.9% (N = 58/70) of surviving patients in this study
group (one died by suicide and one died of other causes) being reassessed
at all eight of these completed follow-up waves.

RELIABILITY SUB-STUDIES

We have also conducted four reliability sub-studies involving the entire
MSAD interview battery. Baseline inter-rater reliability was assessed using
45 conjoint interviews, while test–retest reliability was assessed using two
separate, blind interviews of 30 subjects. We also assessed two different
forms of inter-rater reliability during the follow-up periods. Follow-up

inter-rater reliability was assessed using 48 conjoint interviews of subjects participating in either their two- or four-year follow-up assessment. Follow-up longitudinal (inter-rater) reliability was assessed using 36 videotaped interviews that were made by first-generation raters and later viewed by second- and third-generation raters.

Good to excellent levels of inter-rater and test–retest reliability were achieved at baseline for both Axis I and II disorders (Zanarini & Frankenburg, 2001a). Good to excellent levels of follow-up inter-rater reliability (between raters of the same study generation) and follow-up longitudinal inter-rater reliability (between baseline and follow-up raters). were also found for Axis I and II disorders over time.

We not only assessed the reliability of the *DSM-III-R* diagnosis of BPD in these four sub-studies (which was consistently found to be greater than .85 and thus, in the excellent range); we also assessed the reliability of the DIB-R diagnosis of BPD, and it, too, was found to be excellent in each of these four reliability sub-studies (Zanarini, Frankenburg, & Vujanovic, 2002). In addition, we assessed the reliability of the 22 symptoms of BPD assessed by the DIB-R. Excellent kappas were found in each of the three inter-rater reliability sub-studies for the vast majority (18 or more) of borderline symptoms assessed by the DIB-R. Test–retest reliability for these symptoms was somewhat lower, but still very good (i.e., a third of the BPD symptoms assessed had a kappa in the excellent range, and the remaining two-thirds had a kappa in the fair–good range. In addition, all five dimensional measures of borderline psychopathology (affect section score, cognition section score, impulse action pattern section score, interpersonal relationship section score, and DIB-R total score) had ICCs (intraclass correlation coefficients) in the excellent range for all four reliability sub-studies.

CONVERGENT VALIDITY OF PSYCHOSOCIAL FUNCTIONING

About one-third of the borderline patients and Axis II comparison subjects (N = 108) were randomly selected during the four-year wave to have an informant (typically a close friend or family member) interviewed concerning their psychosocial functioning using a modified version of the BFI-R (Zanarini, Frankenburg, Hennen, et al., 2005). High levels of convergent validity were found. More specifically, a rho value of .92 was found for vocational variables, .83 for relationship variables, and .59 for variables assessing leisure time activities.

BASELINE FINDINGS

This sample of borderline patients reported difficulties in many areas, ranging from troubled family backgrounds to self-mutilation.

Childhood Adversity

Most of this sample of borderline patients reported coming from troubled backgrounds. Over 90% reported some type of abuse in childhood and over 90% reported some type of neglect before the age of 18 (Zanarini et al., 1997). In terms of abuse, 62% reported a childhood history of sexual abuse, and 86% reported a childhood history of verbal, emotional, and/or physical abuse. Most of those reporting a childhood history of sexual abuse reported being severely sexually abused (i.e., over 75% reported abuse that was ongoing and/or involved penetration) (Zanarini, Yong, et al., 2002). In addition, the severity of childhood sexual abuse, other forms of abuse, and neglect were all significantly correlated to both severity of borderline psychopathology and severity of psychosocial impairment.

High percentages of borderline patients also reported being abused and neglected by caretakers of both genders (Zanarini, Frankenburg, Reich, Marino, et al., 2000). More specifically, over 50% reported a childhood history of biparental abuse, and over 70% reported a childhood history of biparental neglect. In addition, the combination of female caretaker neglect and male caretaker abuse was found to be a risk factor for childhood sexual abuse by a non-caretaker for women with BPD.

Borderline patients were also significantly more likely to remember childhood difficulties with separation than Axis II comparison subjects (Reich & Zanarini, 2001). In addition, they were significantly more likely to report more mood reactivity and poorer frustration tolerance in childhood than Axis II comparison subjects.

Family History of Psychiatric Disorder

As noted, family history of psychiatric disorder was also studied in this sample (Zanarini, Frankenburg, Yong, et al., 2004). It was found that the first-degree relatives of borderline patients had a heightened prevalence of *DSM-III-R* and *DSM-IV* BPD. It was also found that they had a heightened prevalence of the symptoms of BPD, particularly inappropriate anger, affective instability, paranoia/dissociation, general impulsivity, and intense, unstable relationships. Not surprisingly, the symptoms of BPD were substantially more common among these relatives than BPD itself.

We also studied the relationship between BPD and other disorders in their first-degree relatives (Zanarini, Barison, Frankenburg, Reich, & Hudson, 2009). Using structural models for familial coaggregation, it was found that BPD coaggregates with major depression, dysthymic disorder, bipolar I disorder, alcohol abuse/dependence, drug abuse/dependence, panic disorder, social phobia, obsessive-compulsive disorder, generalized anxiety disorder, post-traumatic stress disorder (PTSD), somatoform pain disorder, and all four Axis II disorders studied. Taken together, the results of this study suggest that common familial factors, particularly in the areas of affective disturbance and impulsivity, contribute to BPD.

Co-occurring Disorders

Both Axis I and II disorders were found to be common among these borderline patients. The most common lifetime Axis I disorders were unipolar mood disorders and anxiety disorders, particularly PTSD, panic disorder, and social phobia (Zanarini, Frankenburg, Dubo, Sickel, Trikha, Levin, & Reynolds, 1998b). Substance use disorders and eating disorders, particularly eating disorder NOS, were also common (Marino & Zanarini, 2001). In terms of Axis II disorders, paranoid PD, avoidant PD, dependent PD, and self-defeating PD were most common (Zanarini et al., 1998a).

Subsyndromal Phenomenology

The subsyndromal phenomenology of BPD was also studied at baseline. It was found that the subjective pain of borderline patients (i.e., dysphoric affective and cognitive states) was both more pervasive and more multi-faceted than previously recognized (Zanarini et al., 1998). For example, 75% of borderline patients reported feeling damaged beyond repair up to 90% of the time.

Dissociation was found to be heterogeneous in severity, with about a third of borderline patients reporting "normal" levels of dissociation, about 40% reporting moderate levels of dissociation, and about a quarter reporting high levels of dissociation typically associated with PTSD or dissociative identity disorder (DID) (Zanarini, Ruser, Frankenburg, & Hennen, 2000). It was also found that borderline patients had elevated levels of absorption (e.g., some people sometimes find that when they are alone they talk out loud to themselves) and amnesia (e.g., some people sometimes find evidence that they have done things that they do not remember doing) as well as depersonalization. In addition, childhood sexual abuse, inconsistent treatment by a caretaker, witnessing sexual violence as a child, and an adult rape history were found to be significant predictors of the level of dissociation (Zanarini, Ruser, Frankenburg, Hennen, & Gunderson, 2000) as measured by the Dissociative Experiences Scale (DES) (Bernstein & Putnam, 1986).

Onset of Self-Mutilation

Age of onset of self-mutilation was also studied during each participant's index admission (Zanarini, Frankenburg, Ridolfi, et al., 2006). Of the 91%

of borderline patients with a history of self-mutilation, 32.8% reported first harming themselves as children (12 or younger), 30.2% as adolescents (13–17 years old), and 37% as adults (18 or older). After controlling for baseline age, it was found that those with a childhood onset reported more episodes of self-harm, a longer duration of self-harm, and a greater number of methods of self-harm. The results of this study suggest that a sizeable minority of borderline patients first engage in self-harm as children, and that the course of their self-mutilation may be particularly malignant. In addition, it is clear that the majority of borderline patients with a history of childhood and adolescent self-mutilation used this type of behavior as a form of self-soothing without any societal cues, as this type of behavior received no media attention during the time period when these people were under the age of 18. However, it is possible that those 18 and older may have learned about this behavior pattern from other patients once they began psychiatric treatment.

Treatment History Prior to Study Entry

By the time of their index admission, a high percentage of borderline patients had a history of psychiatric treatment (Zanarini, Frankenburg, Khera, et al., 2001). Over three-quarters had been in individual therapy, had previous psychiatric hospitalizations, and been on standing medications. In addition, more than 50% had participated in self-help groups. About 35–45% had been in group therapy, couples/family therapy, day treatment, and residential treatment. Only electroconvulsive therapy (ECT) was rare among borderline patients (<10%).

Prospective Assessment over Time

We have also examined these and additional areas of psychopathology and functioning over time. We first examined the six-year course of BPD. In retrospect, we probably viewed these first longitudinal findings in too optimistic a light, as we focused on the many changes in a positive direction. We next examined the 10-year course of BPD, and by this time, we began to notice areas with a more guarded prognosis, particularly vocational functioning and physical health. We next examined the first 16 years of prospective follow-up, and these analyses revealed what might be viewed as sub-types or sub-groups of those with BPD: those who achieved a concurrent symptomatic remission and good social and good full-time vocational functioning (recovered borderline patients), vs. those who did not (non-recovered borderline patients). The following chapters will describe our findings over these waves of prospective assessment.

5

The Symptoms of Borderline Personality Disorder Assessed in MSAD

STUDY CRITERIA SETS

Patients had to meet both the Revised Diagnostic Interview for Borderlines (DIB-R) (Zanarini, Gunderson, Frankenburg, et al., 1989) and the *DSM-III-R* criteria sets for BPD to be included in the borderline study group. As is well known, the *DSM-III-R* criteria set for BPD consists of eight symptoms, and a cutoff of five symptoms is required to be given the diagnosis. The DIB-R assesses 22 symptoms. It is divided into four sections: affects, cognitions, impulsive acts, and interpersonal symptoms. A score of eight out of ten for the entire interview is required for the diagnosis.

Box 5.1 details the eight *DSM-III-R* criteria for BPD. As can be seen, three are affective (affective instability, intense anger, and chronic feelings of emptiness or boredom), one is cognitive (serious identity disturbance), two are impulsive (self-mutilation/suicide threats/suicide attempts and two other forms of impulsivity), and the other two are interpersonal

Box 5.1 *DSM-III-R* CRITERIA FOR BORDERLINE PERSONALITY DISORDER

A pervasive pattern of instability of mood, interpersonal relationships, and self-image, beginning by early adulthood and present in a variety of contexts, as indicated by at least five of the following:

(1) A pattern of unstable and intense interpersonal relationships characterized by alternating between extremes of overidealization and devaluation

(2) Impulsiveness in at least two areas that are potentially self-damaging, e.g., spending, sex, substance use, shoplifting, reckless driving, binge eating

(3) Affective instability: marked shifts from baseline mood to depression, irritability, or anxiety, usually lasting a few hours and only rarely more than a few days

(4) Inappropriate, intense anger or lack of control of anger, e.g., frequent displays of temper, constant anger, recurrent physical fights

(5) Recurrent suicidal threats, gestures, or behavior, or self-mutilating behavior

(6) Marked and persistent identity disturbance manifested by uncertainty about at least two of the following: self-image, sexual orientation, long-term goals or career choice, type of friends desired, preferred values

(7) Chronic feelings of emptiness or boredom

(8) Frantic efforts to avoid real or imagined abandonment

(frantic efforts to avoid real or imagined abandonment, and intense and unstable relationships).

Table 5.1 lists the 24 symptoms studied—22 from the DIB-R and two from the *DSM-III-R* criteria set not covered by the DIB-R—affective instability and serious identity disturbance. Affective instability, as noted, is an

TABLE 5.1 DIB-R AND *DSM-III-R* SYMPTOMS OF BPD STUDIED

Affective Features	**Interpersonal Features**
Chronic/major depression	Intolerance of aloneness
Chronic feelings of helplessness/	Abandonment/engulfment/annihilation
hopelessness/worthlessness/guilt	concerns
Chronic anger/frequent angry acts	Counterdependency/serious conflict over
	help/care
Chronic anxiety	Stormy relationships
Chronic loneliness/emptiness	Dependency/masochism
Cognitive Features	Devaluation/manipulation/sadism
Odd thinking/unusual perceptual	Demandingness/entitlement
experiences	Treatment regressions
Non-delusional paranoia	Countertransference problems/"special
Quasi-psychotic thought	treatment relationships"
Impulsive Features	***DSM-III-R* Criteria for BPD Not**
	Assessed by DIB-R
Substance abuse/dependence	Affective instability
Sexual deviance (mostly promiscuity)	Serious identity disturbance
Self-mutilation	
Manipulative suicide efforts	
Other (miscellaneous) impulsive	
patterns (e.g., spending sprees,	
shoplifting, reckless driving)	

affective symptom, and serious identity disturbance is seen as a cognitive symptom as it comprises overvalued or basically untrue ideas of inner badness. However, before reporting on the course of these symptoms over time, it is important to describe their clinical importance and their inner meaning to borderline patients.

Before detailing the course of these symptoms, we will describe them in more depth. We will review the affective and cognitive symptoms we studied, as well as self-destructive forms of impulsivity and outmoded interpersonal survival strategies that we studied. Our goal is to provide a more accurate picture of BPD and a more sympathetic portrait of this most challenging and painful disorder.

SECTORS OF PSYCHOPATHOLOGY

Below is a description of the four sectors of borderline psychopathology studied.

Chronic and Intense Dysphoria

Borderline patients suffer from a range of intense dysphoric affects (Gunderson & Kolb, 1978; Zanarini, Gunderson, & Frankenburg, 1990). These affects include depression and sorrow, anger and rage, anxiety and panic, feelings of helplessness, hopelessness, and worthlessness, and feelings of emptiness and loneliness. What distinguishes borderline patients from other patient groups, as noted before, is the number of dysphoric affects they feel at the same time and the overall amplitude of this pain (Zanarini, Frankenburg, DeLuca, et al., 1998).

It is difficult to know what causes these varied and shifting affects. It may be that they are the result of or the sequelae of "kindling events," such as childhood experiences of a traumatic nature (for a review of this literature, see Chapter 2). Alternatively, they may represent a segment of the underlying hyperbolic temperament that we have suggested is core to the borderline diagnosis (Zanarini & Frankenburg 1994) (see Chapter 2 for a more detailed description of this type of temperament). It may also be that these dysphoric affects are due to some type of biological dysfunction. For example, the results of biochemical studies have typically found reduced serotonergic activity in criteria-defined borderline patients (Coccaro et al., 1989; Hollander et al., 1994). In reality, these factors are not totally separate; thus, the tendency toward intense dysphoria may be due to a combination of all three factors.

One of the most difficult aspects of the dysphoria of borderline patients is that treaters often feel compelled to try to lessen its intensity or to eliminate it. Clearly, the problem with this is that no medication is going to "cure" someone of BPD, and it may not even affect the target symptom at which it is aimed. Another reaction is to mistake the dysphoria (and the lability) of borderline patients for any one of a number of comorbid conditions (Zanarini et al., 1998b). This is a problem, as it leaves many aspects of BPD untreated, particularly those of an interpersonal and a temperamental nature. Additionally, it often comes as a surprise to these treaters how treatment-resistant these symptoms are. This may lead to heroic efforts to medicate away what is really the patient's "dis-ease." Clearly, patients who do not feel that people care about them or hear them are not going to be happy that someone, however well intentioned, is trying to take away their pain. In response to these efforts, borderline patients may develop other symptoms or seem to have their Axis I pathology transformed into yet another disorder.

The best approach to dealing with this type of intense and shifting dysphoria is to empathize with how hard it is to deal with these feelings and to acknowledge the likelihood that they will persist, to one degree or another, for the foreseeable future. This lets the patient know that others are aware of her suffering. It also helps to reassure the severely ill borderline patient who typically is fearful that her pain will both never end, and end too soon. This does not mean that medications should not be used if these feelings escalate into a treatable Axis I disorder. It does mean that grief will probably not yield to pharmacotherapy, and as in treating other bereaved patients, patience is more likely to win the day than aggressive polypharmacy.

Cognitive Problems

Borderline patients suffer from three levels of cognitive symptomatology: troubling but nonpsychotic problems, such as overvalued ideas of worthlessness and guilt, experiences of depersonalization and derealization, and nondelusional suspiciousness and ideas of reference; quasi-psychotic or psychotic-like symptoms (i.e., transitory, circumscribed, and somewhat reality-based delusions and hallucinations); and genuine or true delusions and hallucinations. The last category is rare and almost always occurs in the context of a psychotic depression (Pope, Jonas, Hudson, Cohen, & Tohen, 1985; Zanarini, Gunderson, & Frankenburg, 1990). The other two categories or levels are ongoing problems for many severely disturbed borderline patients. The literature is contradictory with regard to the issue of whether these symptoms are trauma-related or not (Brodsky, Cloitre, & Dulit, 1995; Shearer, 1994; Zanarini, Ruser, Frankenburg, Hennen, & Gunderson, 2000; Zweig-Frank, Paris, & Guzder, 1994a, 1994b). The best evidence seems to suggest that most severely disturbed borderline patients suffer from these symptoms, but that these symptoms are more intense in borderline patients reporting childhood histories of sexual abuse. Thus, they seem both intrinsic to the disorder and stress-related.

As for managing these symptoms, the cognitive distortions implicit in overvalued ideas can be explored. Clearly, it is not uncommon for those who have been the object of some type of neglect and/or abuse, however subtle or commonplace, to blame themselves for what has gone wrong in their lives and the lives of those they love and on whom they depend. Their suspiciousness also may have a basis in reality. When the high rates of childhood abuse and neglect reported by borderline patients in ten studies were unknown (Herman et al., 1989; Links, Steiner, & Offord, 1988; Ogata et al., 1990; Paris et al., 1994a; Paris et al., 1994b; Salzman et al., 1993; Shearer et al., 1990; Westen et al., 1990; Zanarini, Gunderson, Marino, et al., 1989; Zanarini, Williams, et al., 1997), and psychodynamic theories posited that the etiology of BPD could be found in subtle problems in parenting, their distrust of others was thought of as a near-psychotic symptom (Masterson, 1972; Adler & Buie, 1979). Today, their mistrust and suspiciousness seem more justified, or at least understandable, and treaters are hopeful that borderline patients can be helped to distinguish between the dangers of their childhood and the probably safer circumstances of adulthood.

Quasi-psychotic symptoms in borderline patients may be related to their belief that they have been abandoned; in this view, the symptoms can be seen as a form of cognitive restitution, providing contact with a loved one whom the patient fears she has lost (Gunderson, 1984). It may also be that the severely disturbed borderline patient is suffering from an unrecognized major depression or is reliving some type of body memory as a consequence of physical and/or sexual abuse or assault that may have occurred in childhood and/or adulthood. It may also be that the patient has learned to signal others that she is worried about her pain's being forgotten by complaining of psychotic or psychotic-like symptoms. This pattern, and the view that these symptoms are acts of restitution, can be handled by pointing out the pattern and its meaning for the patient. They can also be helped by adding more support and structure to the patient's life. The severely ill borderline patient will not abandon these symptoms easily or quickly, but at least they will be able to be discussed. Body memories can be normalized by letting the patient know that they are common among adults who have been abused or neglected in severe ways. Quasi-psychotic experiences related to depression may need to be treated with medication. However, it is clear that all of these factors may be at play in the sort of psychotic symptoms exhibited by severely disturbed borderline patients, and an approach that combines useful new information, more support, and possibly, medications, will be necessary.

Problems with Impulsivity

Below is a discussion of various specific forms of impulsivity studied.

SELF-MUTILATION

Self-mutilation in borderline patients is both an unusual form of self-soothing, and an indirect, though very effective, manner of expressing rage. It goes against everything therapists believe in and is often mistakenly taken as a personal affront. This is, in part, the way the patient intends it. But in a larger sense, it is meant to protect the therapist (and others whom the patient loves and needs) from the ravages of the patient's rage and self-hatred; a rage and self-hatred that is truly excoriating. While borderline patients cut and burn themselves because they are dissociated and need to feel "real" and because they need to relieve a tremendous amount of anxiety, they also hurt themselves as a way of managing a murderous degree of frustration and rage. Rather than wasting time feeling upset or even horrified, therapists wishing to work with severely disturbed borderline patients need to remember that in many cases, this type of behavior began in childhood, and at that time, it had nothing to do with treatment and was done in secret. Rather than seeing self-harm as an iatrogenic form of behavior with all of its meaning tied to treatment, it is probably more accurate to see it as a long-standing form of self-soothing; a protective reflexing back onto oneself of volcanic rage; and as an addiction, with all the power that that implies. As one 22-year-old borderline patient said: "I plan to give up my eating disorder when I turn 30, smoking when I turn 40, and cutting and burning when I turn 50. At least I'm trying, aren't I?"

The therapist's first task is to empathize with the pain that led to self-injurious behavior, while the second task is to make it plain to the patient that the therapist will not struggle with the patient over her self-mutilating efforts. If the self-harm is medically insignificant, the patient should take care of it herself or see a general or emergency room physician. However, if the self-harm is medically serious and the patient cannot control it, the previously discussed and mutually agreed upon plan that has arisen during the course of the treatment is to briefly hospitalize the patient. Once there, she can have time to think and cool down, a medication and therapy consultation can take place, and the patient and her therapist can have a brief but needed respite from one another. The third thing to do is to act in a respectful manner toward this powerfully addictive form of behavior. Much as alcoholics do not give up drinking until they are ready, borderline patients will not give up self-mutilation until they have found something or someone who can give them more of the comfort they need and crave. Much as adolescents cannot be cajoled into growing up faster because it is more convenient for their parents, borderline patients cannot be nagged into giving up a form of self-soothing than can be both physically agonizing and the source of feelings of euphoria. This should be one of the goals of treatment, not a precondition for undertaking such a venture.

SUICIDALITY

Many borderline patients threaten suicide on a regular basis when they are worried about being abandoned (Gunderson, 1984). Others make numerous suicide gestures. Serious attempts are not infrequent. And anywhere between 3% and 10% of borderline patients with a history of being hospitalized at least once go on to commit suicide in the long-term follow-up studies described in Chapter 3 (McGlashan 1986; Paris et al., 1987; Stone 1990).

The treater of a seriously disturbed borderline patient needs to take a careful history of the patient's suicidality; both threats and efforts. If a patient is prone to suicide threats but has no history of gestures or attempts, a useful approach is to ask what she thought she was conveying by saying: "If my mother isn't more understanding in the future, I am going to take the family gun and shoot myself at Thanksgiving dinner." This borderline patient may believe she was talking about her frustrations with her mother and not realize that she was subtly shifting responsibility for her anger from herself to the listener, typically her therapist. Often a psychoeducational approach that lets the patient "hear" how she sounds and that provides her with alternative ways of expressing her feelings will be very helpful, if not openly appreciated.

Much the same approach can be taken with the borderline patient who takes several aspirins and then presents at an emergency room, or cuts herself with a plastic knife and hopes to die. However, a very different approach needs to be taken with the borderline patient with a history of serious suicide attempts. Often such a patient will have a striking history of mood disorder (typically unipolar), an ongoing substance abuse problem, and a family history of suicidality. All three of these factors need to be taken into account when contingency plans are being made. When dealing with this triad of risk factors, the treater should encourage the patient to get aggressive treatment for both her mood disorder and her substance abuse. All too often, treaters overlook a borderline patient's emerging major depression because it arises insidiously out of her chronic dysphoria. And time and again, therapists make far too little of their borderline patient's drinking problem or abuse of prescription or street medications. Clearly, they need to get clean and sober and stay that way until their life is under better control. It is not uncommon for borderline patients who episodically abused alcohol or drugs (typically marijuana) during their late teens or early twenties to be able to drink socially or occasionally use drugs recreationally. However, chronic abusers need to seek out specialized treatment for their substance abuse problems (e.g., Linehan's treatment aimed at decreasing drug abuse among borderline women [Linehan et al., 1999]). Only after sobriety is achieved and maintained for a substantial amount of time should a more traditional psychotherapy be undertaken. In addition, lifetime sobriety must be a goal for these patients. Some might disagree with these recommendations and suggest treating BPD and all comorbid disorders concurrently. In some ways, this makes sense. However, few patients, in our experience, have the emotional bandwidth or the finances to devote all of their time to recovery from this cluster of serious illnesses.

Another important approach to the borderline patient with a history of deep and prolonged depressions that have been associated with serious suicide attempts is to empathize with the difficulty of managing such a serious illness on top of all of her other problems. It is both frightening and discouraging to both patient and treater that depressive episodes keep recurring and that they may be deeper and more prolonged as time goes by. Often, simply having a treater address the implications of having a personal and family history of depression and suicidality will be a relief to a borderline patient. Relentlessly looking for interpersonally based precipitating factors and encouraging her to believe that one day she will no longer have to worry about being depressed may only be making her feel more discouraged and alone. It may well be that she will not get depressed again if all goes well for her, but it may be liberating to share the possibility that this is a lifelong struggle and one in which mental health professionals treating the patient are prepared to participate.

Clearly, there is no known way of predicting which seriously ill borderline patients will commit suicide. Plainly, it is a bad prognostic sign if a family member has tried or succeeded in killing him- or herself. To the patient, this represents the breaking of a taboo, such that what was once unthinkable now enters the realm of the acceptable.

Oftentimes a seriously ill borderline patient will begin to play a game of "cat and mouse" with her therapist (and with her own life) around the issue of suicidality. What can and should be done in such a situation? Termination always comes to mind and may realistically be an option if carried out in an appropriate and ethical manner. Bringing other people onto the treatment team, getting a consultation, and persuading the patient to live in a residential center is probably more helpful. It is also important to talk with such a patient about the real possibility that she will die as a result of all of her suicidal efforts, and to let her know that you would miss her, although your life will certainly go on. Although some clinicians might feel uncomfortable with this degree of self-disclosure, our experience suggests that most severely disturbed borderline patients have no idea of the affection and respect in which they are held. On the other hand, it is important to address any misconceptions about who would actually be dying by reminding the patient that any vengeful feelings she has toward her therapist or other members of the treatment team will only be very partially satisfied. If the patient has children, you may also want to discuss with her how her death might affect them, particularly given her own knowledge of the pain of being abandoned. In the most refractory of circumstances, anticipatory mourning (or a deeply felt acknowledgement by patient and therapist alike of the grief that is sure to accompany suicide) may help to alleviate some of the desperation driving such a patient. It also allows the therapist to come to grips with this very real possibility and may even help the patient's family accept that death may be on the horizon for their child.

Interpersonal Problems

Below is a description of specific interpersonal problems that are commonly manifested by patients with BPD.

DEVALUATION

Devaluation has been viewed as one of the primary defenses of borderline patients (Kernberg, 1967); or, alternatively, as a particularly annoying
form of "misbehavior" by many clinicians. In reality, if properly understood, devaluation is useful for patient and treater alike—at least in the
initial stages of treatment. The value of devaluation is that the borderline
patient uses it to negotiate intimacy, albeit in a very awkward manner.
After all, no one bothers to put someone down unless they are emotionally important to them in some way. Borderline patients are affiliative by
nature and wish to be close to others, but are hindered in their quest for
closeness by their fears of being unwanted or used.

Devaluation is also potentially useful for the treater in that it is a window
into the patient's own extraordinarily low self-esteem. Devaluation is an
emotionally taxing but still useful crash course in what the borderline patient tends to feel on a day-to-day basis. In our experience, devaluation is
learned while young, much like other overlearned forms of behavior. And
much like other forms of overlearned behavior, the borderline patient is
oblivious to the actual content of her behavior and its effects on others.
This is so because the families of many borderline patients expressed their
love and devotion in a "biting," indirect manner; and thus, the borderline
patient is not fully and consistently aware that implying or stating that
someone is stupid, mean, or completely unhelpful engenders hurt feelings
in friends and treaters alike.

It is as though borderline patients speak a special language, and treaters
must learn to translate this language rapidly for the therapeutic relationship to proceed with a certain degree of smoothness and emotional tone.
Thus, a borderline patient may say: "No one loves me or listens to me.
No one cares." The therapist, who is meeting with the patient at 7:00 in
the evening and feeling tired and hungry, can take this comment personally and angrily confront the patient with her lack of gratitude. Or
he can quickly translate this verbal missive into what the patient actually
meant. This process of translation allows the treater to respond to what
the patient thought she said with a careful clarification that protects the
patient's fragile self-esteem while providing the patient with useful new

information in a manner that she can actually "hear." Such a clarification might be: "Sometimes people find it hard to let people know that they care for them." This type of comment gives the borderline patient time and room to think about her behavior without being criticized for it. It is put somewhat in the third person and directed at the middle distance. It, or a variant of it, will have to be repeated many times on many occasions before the borderline patient seems to "get it." However, it is our clinical experience that even the most severely disturbed borderline patient has typically noted this comment from the beginning, thought about it often, but will not acknowledge it or its usefulness until the desperation that underlies devaluation has abated.

MANIPULATION

Most borderline patients are highly skilled at manipulation, which we define here as trying to get what one wants from others in an indirect manner. Needs are not directly expressed, and wishes are not completely owned. Rather, borderline patients try to maneuver people in much the same manner as small children put their mother's hand in the cookie jar when they are hungry for a snack. Much as children "use" their mother because they are small and relatively weak and powerless, borderline patients try to take from people that which might ordinarily be freely and openly given, or at least refused in a polite and respectful manner. But treaters often take manipulation personally and respond by trying to control or "set limits" with borderline patients. This is so because manipulation is both a felt assault on one's generosity and a seeming indictment of one's naïveté. Many therapists find the borderline patient's propensity to try to manipulate them demeaning and hateful (as well as unnecessary), particularly as they have worked so hard to give up these "uncivil and childish" forms of behavior themselves.

Here again, as with devaluation, borderline patients are unaware of the maladaptive aspects of their behavior and take a confrontation on their manipulativeness as an assault on their right to live. It is far better to use a clarification aimed at the middle ground between patient and treater: "It is hard for some people to believe that they can ever get anything they want." Plainly, most people do not steal food at a buffet dinner. Nor do most hosts get angry at a guest who mistakes a finger bowl for a glass of water. However, treaters often get so angry and outraged at a borderline patient's manipulative behavior that they respond with a chilly superego stance that has more in common with Cotton Mather than Sigmund Freud. Borderline people, like other people stuck in the awkward behavior of adolescence, will respond better to a psychoeducational approach than to a clerical edict. After all, most of us learn more effectively while sitting in a comfortable chair than while trapped in a walk-in refrigerator.

DEMANDINGNESS

Borderline patients often are very insistent about getting what they want when they want it. This behavior is often taken as an affront by their overly civilized therapists, who have worked hard to get what they want by asking politely and waiting patiently. In this view, demandingness is both boorish and embarrassingly obvious. Less experienced therapists often cringe in horror at these naked demands, while quietly wondering if there is something to this brazen, if annoying, approach. More experienced therapists often intuitively realize that only the weak and powerless demand, while the powerful only need ask.

Here, too, a psychoeducational approach is useful, as is an admiring view of the patient's "prowess." One might comment: "Good for you. You are finally taking care of yourself." Or alternatively, one might say: "It's hard to believe that polite people ever get anything." Certainly, borderline patients have been told repeatedly by their family and their previous treaters that demandingness is off-putting. But rarely is this behavior accepted as a way station on the road to true assertiveness. While their false power should not be allowed to rule the day, their efforts at being assertive should be encouraged. This is an important goal in the work with severely disturbed borderline patients, as they are often timid and self-defeating, while at the same time, they rarely go unnoticed due to their insistent bravado.

ENTITLEMENT

To most therapists, entitlement is the evil sister of demandingness. In this view, entitlement is the inner state that underlies demanding behavior. Borderline patients are seen as believing that they have a "divine" right to everything they want, and that the "rules of life" do not apply to them. In many ways, this perception is true. However, in our experience, it is important to remember that the more "entitled" the borderline patient, the more likely she is to be starving herself because she believes that she does not deserve to eat, or cutting herself because she thinks that she is bad or evil.

In many ways, what borderline patients feel entitled to is life the way it used to be before everything went wrong. Or life the way it should have been if everything had not always, in their perception, been wrong. Like most grieving people, borderline patients are obsessed with the past and are unable to let go. The more depleted they feel, the more they believe that only the impossible will make them whole. Thus, borderline patients who have been abused as small children want to be treated in the endlessly loving way that they believe attentive mothers treat their toddlers. Or borderline patients who were neglected when young want an always available parental figure who is never tired, sad, or frustrated.

Much as latency-age children long to be the child of a famous person, borderline patients feel that they deserve the childhood they never had. And so they do. But reality dictates that dead people cannot live again, and childhood is reserved for the very young. The job of a therapist of a severely disturbed borderline patient is not to attack her for her heartfelt wish to be cared for in a loving and tender manner, but to mourn with her the simple fact that the emotional carousel only goes around once for each of us. However, it is also the job of the therapist of the severely disturbed borderline patient to point out that life offers many kinds of reparations but that these disguised adult substitutes can only be found in the real world and are not hidden in the therapist's office in some emotional toy chest that only the lucky few get to open. Neither persistence nor insistence will bring back the childhood one never had.

TREATMENT REGRESSIONS

Just when a therapist feels that he or she has done a particularly good piece of therapeutic work, the severely borderline patient may undergo a serious regression in outpatient treatment. Typically, there are two reasons for this. The first is that the therapist has, or the patient believes that the therapist has, inadvertently "promised" the patient more than he or she can or will deliver. In this situation, the patient's hopes for a perfect relationship have been raised only to be dashed and the patient feels profoundly embarrassed, betrayed, and enraged. And like anyone about to lose their spot in first class, borderline patients hang on for all they are worth. Unfortunately for the therapist, they hang on with all the maladaptive survival skills they have at their command, and the therapeutic relationship can soon take on the appearance of a battlefield strewn with the innocent being punished by the terrified.

The second reason that a serious behavioral regression can occur in outpatient treatment is that the borderline patient believes that she is making too much progress in the real world and that her therapist now believes that she is "all better." Given the centrality of their emotional pain to their sense of themselves (Zanarini & Frankenburg, 1994), this can seem like an affront to all that the severely disturbed borderline patient holds most dear. And like a small child with a new brother or sister, lessons recently learned can be abandoned in the desperate emotional struggle that ensues. This emotional recrudescence of their abandonment fears can unleash a panic and rage that cannot be controlled in an outpatient setting.

This, of course, may lead to an inpatient stay, which may eventually lead to an even more profound behavioral regression. When cornered and made to feel powerless, the severely ill borderline patient may fight back and end up hurting herself to get back a sense of control (Gunderson, 1984). Or alternatively, she may become despairing and abandon all pretense of control and end up in seclusion and restraints. Clearly, few of us do our best learning when tied up and tied down. And for severely disturbed borderline patients, this type of experience may reenact child-hood experiences of physical and/or sexual abuse.

Much as competent therapists do not offer needy borderline patients an unlimited spending spree at an emotional toy store, a well-run inpatient unit does not put a borderline patient in restraints for countertransferentially driven reasons, such as "she said she was unsafe" or "she got really angry and I thought she might lose control." Much of the chaos on an inpatient unit trying to work with a borderline patient arises from the inner feelings of the patient that she is being controlled or she has lost all control, and is again small and powerless.

However, a large measure of the chaos arises because so many young people—patients and staff alike—are trapped in a small physical space, with all of their conflicted longings to be taken care of and to take care of others casually intermingled (Main, 1957; Burnham, 1966). In such a situation, borderline patients are going to notice that some staff members are warm and nurturing, and others are more distant and con-trolling. Soon, through the magic of projective identification, these staff members are quarreling with one another over their basic worth. In the end, the severely ill borderline patient will be punished in some way for being inconsiderate enough to notice the real differences in attitudes that always exist on an inpatient unit. She will be seen as deliberately "splitting" staff, and nurses and mental health workers alike will have forgotten that, much as it takes two to tango, it takes two (or more) to engender a regression. Put another way, it is hard to imagine a border-line patient bothering to regress on a desert island. After all, regression is both an awkward and an indirect form of communication, as much as an act of desperation.

While both patient and therapist or inpatient staff are usually implicated in some way when a treatment regression occurs, it is also possible and even probable that the patient has experienced an upsurge in Axis I psy-chopathology that is autonomous. Much as sometimes a cigar is really just a cigar, often a depression is just a constitutionally driven vulnera-bility gone awry. And it is difficult to overestimate the degree to which a

serious major depressive episode can exacerbate already existing borderline psychopathology.

SPECIAL RELATIONSHIPS

As we have said in many places in this chapter, borderline patients long
for a warm and loving relationship with a generous and kindhearted
mother figure. They may also long to recapture the "special" but inappropriate and/or unhelpful relationship that they once had with a
parent or parental figure. Both of these factors make them vulnerable
to both unwitting and predatory therapists. The unwitting therapist
may believe that all the severely ill borderline patient needs is to be re-
parented. Often this belief goes hand-in-hand with the belief that the
patient is not really borderline but rather suffering from a chronic form
of PTSD, and that all of her problems are due to a childhood history
of abuse.

However, what this evangelical therapist forgets or overlooks is that the
borderline patient is far more in need of the lessons most people learn
in latency and adolescence, rather than the emotional swaddling clothes
of early childhood. As Maltsberger and Buie (1974) have pointed out,
such emotionally tender psychotherapeutic trysts are often followed by
enraged reenactments. This is so because borderline patients, no matter
what their wishes, are not infants and know in some deep and pervasive
way that they are not nearly as appealing when balled up in a corner of a
quiet room at the age of 25 as they were when they were taking a nap in
the back of the family car at the age of two.

While experiences of too much giving and then an angry retrench-
ment are common when treating borderline patients, actual friendships
and love affairs between borderline patients and their treaters can be cata-
strophic for all the reasons that incest is so destructive. Love affairs are by
definition mutual and reciprocal. Borderline patients, while they certainly
need supportive life partners, need their therapist as a guide to the rules of
life, not the disappointments of love.

DEPENDENCY AND COUNTERDEPENDENCY

Borderline patients are typically very dependent and prone to helping others at the same time. Their counterdependency can be seen as shame over normal wishes to be taken care of and a deeply held belief that their dependency needs will not be met. It may also be seen as more adaptive and a personality trend that may someday evolve into altruism. In this regard, Vaillant (1977) has found that creativity and generosity are the only two highly adaptive orientations that people with a very troubled childhood are likely to achieve. And thus, this trend should be encouraged in borderline patients. However, they will encounter special difficulties in entering the helping professions, and their potential for envy-driven regressions will need to be anticipated and addressed. Clearly, it is very difficult to help others if one is hungry for help oneself.

The dependency of borderline patients often joins with their desperation to lead them to request or demand more contact with their therapist than is easy or appropriate to give. Sometimes therapists succumb to these demands and end up exhausted and resentful. Other times they set very firm "limits" on their availability. Unfortunately, these limits are often set in such a way that they imply that the patient is misbehaving and needs to be controlled.

Our experience is that it is more helpful to teach borderline patients about boundaries. These are areas that they draw around their own space and time. As so many borderline patients did not learn about the most appropriate interpersonal distances as children, and vacillate between clinging and fleeing behaviors, this can be a useful set of lessons. It also puts the issue under the patient's control and protects her dignity. In addition, it makes it clear that the attainment and maintenance of appropriate boundaries is as much for her sake as for the treater's.

This is not to say that there should be no limitations on the therapy or the demands that a therapist can and should fulfill. Clearly, patients should attend all of their appointments, come on time, leave when scheduled, make some effort, no matter how awkward, to discuss what is actually going on in their lives, and pay their bills in full. Usually problems arise as much because of a therapist's guilt and his or her countertransferential absorption of the patient's abandonment fears, as because of the unrealistic demands that a severely disturbed borderline patient makes. Put another way, therapists treating these patients need to give themselves permission to sleep through the night and to enlist the help of others when a particular patient is putting more strain on them than can reasonably be borne. However, this type of freedom requires that a therapist know that he or she may be operating on the patient's "borrowed" fears, and that neither of them will die as a result of acknowledging their separate identities.

Modern technology also provides treaters with help in dealing with the borderline patient's wish for frequent extra-session contact. Email is a useful tool in this regard, as are texts. Voice mail is also useful in providing borderline patients with the contact they crave and perhaps need due to their problems with object constancy (Adler & Buie, 1979). Voice mail allows them to call at all hours, listen to their therapist's voice, and in this way, restabilize themselves. It also allows them the opportunity to record, replay, and then erase angry messages to which they do not want their therapist to listen. This process, while initially secret, typically finds its way into therapy and can then be discussed in a useful way.

DISTORTIONS OF THE TRUTH RELATED
TO SERIOUS IDENTITY DISTURBANCE

Borderline patients often lie, or at least tell different people different versions of their truth. While some borderline patients have strong sociopathic tendencies, the majority do not. Rather, they "lie" for three reasons. The first reason is to bolster their shaky sense of self by coming up with a personal truth that is more bearable to them and perhaps more appealing to others. In this regard, they may be boastful and claim accomplishments that are not really theirs. The second reason is that they are particularly afraid of disappointing others and/or being punished for being less than perfect. Thus, they bend the truth, often through critical omissions, to avoid losing the support of those they care about and trust. The third reason for their tendency to make misrepresentations is that they do not know what the shared or objective truth is. This can be due to their varied and shifting sense of identity. It can also be due to the fact that treaters have been so insistent that abuse is at the root of all of their problems, even if they disagree, that they no longer have a personal narrative in which they believe and from which they derive a sense of continuity and identity.

A useful approach when dealing with this tendency is for the therapist to consistently point out the inconsistencies in what the patient is telling him or her. This will put the patient on notice that others pay attention to what she is saying and hold her accountable for at least trying to make sense in a shared manner. The second useful approach is not crowding the patient with an externally imposed version of the truth of her life, but instead listening carefully as she develops or, more probably, simply relates a personal narrative she has been quietly, even secretly, working on for years.

SADOMASOCHISTIC TENDENCIES (MASOCHISM AND SADISM)

Borderline patients often alternate between behaving like a victim and victimizing others. They are both submissive and controlling by nature and experience. Therapists are quick to notice how cruelly they can behave, and therapists rightly resent trying to be controlled or treated in a cruel manner. Here, too, they are likely to react by reinforcing or imposing overly strict "limits." When using this approach, they often end up with a more compliant patient or no patient at all, as borderline patients often prematurely terminate treatment when their feelings are hurt too deeply.

Therapists are not as good, in our experience, at noticing how masochistic their severely disturbed borderline patients are. When angry and frustrated enough, therapists can overlook the self-destructive aspects of many behaviors, such as bingeing and purging, having unprotected sex, and routinely driving at 95 miles per hour. They can also come to view self-mutilation and even very serious suicide attempts as forms of misbehavior meant only or mainly to ruin the therapist's evening, weekend, or vacation. Clearly in this situation, the therapist is out of touch with his or her own cruelty and has come to view the patient as all bad. Such simplistic thinking is dangerous when treating severely ill borderline patients as it reinforces their sense of their own inner badness. A more useful approach is to refuse to struggle with them or to try to avoid attempts to control them. Rather, an educational approach points out how it is in the patients' interest to take care of themselves and not alienate others by treating them in the unfortunate way that the patients remember being treated. Often, appeals to self-interest and the hopeful power of the Golden Rule ("Do unto others as you would have them do unto you") are effective tools when working with a severely disturbed borderline patient.

CONCLUSIONS

Severely ill borderline patients are among the most challenging in the field of mental health. Often they have suffered deeply as children and developed a series of symptoms and behaviors that helped them survive while young, but that limit them as adults. Clinicians wishing to work with these patients need to have an optimistic nature, a good sense of humor, and an iron constitution. Common sense is probably a more important tool for their treaters to possess than a wish to conduct a sophisticated empirically-based psychotherapy.

While many clinicians view such patients with anxious dread, we suggest that one can admire the integrity with which they have dealt with their pain. After all, not many people remain so loyal to and so respectful of disheartening experiences engendered by their temperament, their environment, or some combination of the two.

6

The Long-Term Course of the Symptoms of Borderline Personality Disorder

BASELINE TO SIX-YEAR FOLLOW-UP

After following this sample of borderline patients and Axis II comparison subjects for six years, we examined the course of the 24 symptoms of BPD that we are studying (Zanarini, Frankenburg, Hennen, et al., 2003). More specifically, we studied the prevalence rates or percentages of both groups reporting each symptom at each time point: baseline, two-year follow-up, four-year follow-up, and six-year follow-up. We found that a significantly higher percentage of borderline patients than Axis II comparison subjects reported or were judged to exhibit each of these 24 symptoms. We also found that the prevalence rates for both study groups declined at about the same rate over time.

Table 6.1 details the prevalence rates for borderline patients at baseline (two years prior to their index admission) and at six-year follow-up (fifth and sixth years after their index admission).

TABLE 6.1   PREVALENCE OF SYMPTOMS OF BPD REPORTED
BY BORDERLINE PATIENTS AT BASELINE AND SIX-YEAR FOLLOW-UP

	Baseline	Six-Year Follow-up
Affective Features		
Chronic/major depression	98.6	70.1
Chronic feelings of helplessness/hopelessness/ worthlessness	98.3	61.0
Chronic anger/frequent angry acts	95.2	79.2
Chronic anxiety	94.5	64.0
Chronic loneliness/emptiness	98.6	72.4
Cognitive Features		
Odd thinking/unusual perceptual experiences	88.3	49.2
Non-delusional paranoia	85.5	56.8
Quasi-psychotic thought	56.6	20.1
Impulsive Features		
Substance abuse/dependence	49.0	25.0
Sexual deviance (mostly promiscuity)	26.9	11.7
Self-mutilation	80.7	28.4
Manipulative suicide efforts	81.4	25.8
Other (miscellaneous) impulsive patterns	93.8	65.5
Interpersonal Features		
Intolerance of aloneness	92.1	67.4
Abandonment/engulfment/annihilation concerns	92.1	64.8
Counterdependency/serious conflict over help/care	95.5	67.8
Stormy relationships	78.3	46.6
Dependency/masochism	92.1	65.2
Devaluation/manipulation/sadism	86.6	40.2
Demandingness/entitlement	62.1	26.9
Treatment regressions	43.8	12.5
Countertransference problems/"special treatment relationships"	47.9	11.4

TABLE 6.1 CONTINUED

	Baseline	Six-Year Follow-up
DSM-III-R Criteria for BPD Not Assessed by DIB-R		
Affective Instability	90.0	50.4
Serious Identity Disturbance	78.6	27.3

The results of this study suggest that different sectors of borderline psychopathology have different longitudinal patterns. The affective symptoms of BPD were the least likely to resolve for borderline patients, affecting 61–79% of borderline patients at six-year follow-up. While this is a very significant decline from the 95–99% rate found at baseline, it indicates that the majority of borderline patients continued to suffer from a range of dysphoric affects. Previously, we detailed the dysphoric states specific to BPD (Zanarini et al., 1998), and the results of this study suggested that many of these states are relatively resistant to change. The clinical implications of this finding are unclear. The majority of borderline patients remained in treatment throughout these follow-up periods (Zanarini, Frankenburg, Hennen, & Silk, 2004); thus, this lack of symptom resolution is probably not due to a failure to treat these symptoms. Rather, it may be that these affective symptoms are core features of a borderline patient's identity or temperament and, as such, are relatively resistant to change. Whether new treatments aimed at this sector of borderline psychopathology can be developed and would prove useful is an open question.

The impulsive symptoms of BPD were the most likely to resolve for borderline patients. Both self-mutilation and suicide efforts were reported by 81% of borderline patients at baseline. By the six-year follow-up, the rates for both of these forms of self-destructive behavior had declined to about 25%. In a like manner, substance abuse declined from a baseline high of 49% to 25% at six-year follow-up, and sexual deviance (mostly promiscuity) had declined from 27% to 12%. In contrast, other forms of impulsivity, which included eating binges, verbal outbursts, and spending sprees, only declined from 94% at baseline to 66% at six-year follow-up.

The cognitive and interpersonal symptoms of BPD occupy an intermediate position in terms of their longitudinal course. While all three cognitive and all nine interpersonal symptom patterns declined significantly over time, some declined to substantially lower levels than others. A history of quasi-psychotic thought was reported by over half of the borderline patients (57%) at baseline, but by six-year follow-up, only 20% reported experiencing such transitory, circumscribed delusions and hallucinations. Both odd thinking/unusual perceptual experiences (mostly overvalued ideas, recurrent illusions, depersonalization, and derealization) and nondelusional paranoia were much more common at baseline, being reported by over 85% of borderline patients. After six years of follow-up, about half of borderline patients (49–57%) still reported these symptoms.

As noted previously, the DIB-R assesses the presence of nine interpersonal symptom patterns. Two of these patterns, treatment regressions and countertransference problems, initially reported by less than 50% of borderline patients, were reported by only about 10% of borderline patients by six-year follow-up. Three other patterns (stormy relationships, devaluation/manipulation/sadism, and demandingness/entitlement) were reported by anywhere from about 60–85% of borderline patients at baseline, and about a quarter to less than half at six-year follow-up. The third group of interpersonal symptoms (intolerance of aloneness, abandonment concerns, counterdependency, and dependency/masochism) was originally reported by over 90% of borderline patients, and over 60% of borderline patients were still reporting these symptoms after six years of prospective follow-up.

Taken together, these results suggest that BPD is a disorder characterized by two distinct types of symptoms. One type—such as self-mutilation, suicide efforts, quasi-psychotic thought, treatment regressions, and countertransference problems—is a manifestation of acute illness. These symptoms, which have been found to be particularly good markers for the borderline diagnosis (Zanarini, Gunderson, Frankenburg, & Chauncey, 1990) and which are often associated with treatment crises and/or the need for hospitalization, seem to resolve relatively quickly over time and were only present in a minority of borderline patients followed for six years. The other type of symptom represents the more temperamental or enduring aspects of BPD. These symptoms, such as chronic feelings of anger or emptiness, suspiciousness, difficulty tolerating aloneness, and abandonment concerns, seemed to be resolving at a slower pace and were still reported by a majority of borderline patients six years after their index admission.

In this "complex" model of borderline psychopathology, acute symptoms, which are seen as akin to the positive symptoms of schizophrenia, seem to resolve relatively rapidly, are the best markers for the disorder, and are often the immediate reason for needing costly forms of treatment, such as psychiatric hospitalizations. In contrast, temperamental symptoms, which are so named because the results of longitudinal studies of temperament have suggested that temperament is innate but not immutable (Costa & McCrea, 1992), seem to resolve more slowly, are not specific to BPD, and are closely associated with ongoing psychosocial impairment. They are also seen as akin to the negative symptoms of schizophrenia. In terms of the 24 symptoms studied, the prevalence of five core BPD symptoms was found to decline with particular rapidity: quasi-psychotic thought, self-mutilation, help-seeking suicide efforts, treatment regressions, and countertransference problems. In contrast, feelings of depression, anger, and loneliness/emptiness were the most stable symptoms.

Table 6.2 lists the symptoms believed to be acute and those that are believed to be temperamental. The results of additional studies of this sample that address this issue are described next.

TABLE 6.2   ACUTE AND TEMPERAMENTAL SYMPTOMS OF BPD

Acute Symptoms	Temperamental Symptoms
Affective instability	Chronic/major depression
Quasi-psychotic thought	Chronic feelings of helplessness/ hopelessness/worthlessness/ guilt
Serious identity disturbance	Chronic anger/frequent angry acts
Substance abuse/dependence	Chronic anxiety
Sexual deviance (mostly promiscuity)	Chronic loneliness/emptiness
Self-mutilation	Odd thinking/unusual perceptual experiences
Manipulative suicide efforts	Non-delusional paranoia
Stormy relationships	Other forms of impulsivity
Devaluation/manipulation/sadism	Intolerance of aloneness
Demandingness/entitlement	Abandonment/engulfment/ annihilation concerns
Treatment regressions	Counterdependency/serious conflict over help/care
Countertransference problems/"special treatment relationships"	Dependency/masochism

SURVIVAL ANALYSES FROM BASELINE TO 10-YEAR FOLLOW-UP

Survival analyses begin with all of the borderline patients and comparison subjects in this study who at baseline reported the 24 symptoms being studied, and track time-to-remission for those in each study group (Zanarini et al., 2007). The percentage of initially symptomatic borderline patients and Axis II comparison subjects who exhibited each of 24 symptoms of BPD continuously throughout the follow-up intervals declined substantially over time, with borderline patients showing a significantly slower time-to-remission for most symptoms than did Axis II comparison subjects. More specifically, borderline patients had a significantly slower time-to-remission than Axis II comparison subjects in 19 of these comparisons.

Two main findings have emerged from this study. The first is that half of the symptoms studied declined so substantially that less than 15% of subjects who exhibited them at baseline still exhibited them at 10-year follow-up. These 12 symptoms encompassed all four sectors of borderline psychopathology detailed in the DIB-R or reflected in the *DSM-III-R* criteria for BPD. In the affective realm, only the *DSM-III-R* criterion of affective instability achieved this rapid a time-to-remission. In the cognitive realm, both quasi-psychotic thought and serious identity disturbance remitted at this rapid a rate. (Identity disturbance, as noted before, was included as a cognitive symptom because it is based on false perceptions of the self, such as "I am bad" or "I am damaged beyond repair.") In terms of forms of impulsivity, substance abuse/dependence, promiscuity, self-mutilation, and help-seeking suicide efforts remitted relatively rapidly. In the interpersonal realm, stormy relationships, devaluation/manipulation/sadism, demandingness/entitlement, serious treatment regressions, and countertransference problems/"special" treatment relationships all remitted relatively quickly.

The second main finding is that the other 12 symptoms studied declined less substantially, with about 20–40% of borderline subjects who exhibited them at baseline still exhibiting them at 10-year follow-up. These 12 symptoms also encompassed all four sectors of borderline psychopathology detailed in the DIB-R. In the affective realm, all five forms of chronic dysphoria studied demonstrated a relatively slow time-to-remission. For example, intense anger was still experienced by over 45% of initially angry borderline patients 10 years after their index admission. In the cognitive realm, both odd thinking/unusual perceptual experiences and nondelusional paranoia were relatively slow to remit. In terms of forms of impulsivity, only general impulsivity, which was most commonly some form of disordered eating, speeding sprees, or reckless driving, remained relatively common after 10 years of prospective follow-up. Four interpersonal symptoms were also relatively slow to remit: intolerance of aloneness, abandonment/

engulfment/annihilation fears, counterdependency, and undue dependency/masochism.

This division makes conceptual sense. More specifically, most acute symptoms either reflect core areas of impulsivity (e.g., self-mutilation, help-seeking suicide efforts) or active attempts to manage interpersonal difficulties (e.g., problems with demandingness/entitlement, serious treatment regressions). In contrast, most temperamental symptoms seem to be either affective symptoms reflecting areas of chronic dysphoria (e.g., anger, loneliness/emptiness) or interpersonal symptoms reflecting abandonment and dependency issues (e.g., intolerance of aloneness, counterdependency problems). Looked at another way, most acute symptoms seem to have an active, even assertive, component, while most temperamental symptoms seem to reflect a certain degree of fearfulness and passivity.

Twice as many symptoms of BPD seemed to resolve with relatively rapidity in our current study as in our previous study of the six-year course of BPD symptoms (Zanarini, Frankenburg, Hennen, et al., 2003). This difference is not surprising, as the current study assesses time-to-remission of symptoms over ten years of prospective follow-up, while our prior study detailed the percentage of patients exhibiting each symptom at baseline and each of three two-year follow-up periods.

CUMULATIVE RATES OF SYMPTOMATIC REMISSION AND RECURRENCE AFTER 16 YEARS OF PROSPECTIVE FOLLOW-UP

After 16 years of prospective follow-up, we studied cumulative rates of symptomatic remissions lasting two years or four years (Zanarini et al., 2016). For the first time, we also studied symptomatic recurrences—after remissions lasting two or four years. Again, survival analyses were used—which begin with the patients reporting a symptom in the two years before their index admission and result in a cumulative total for each symptom of the percent who have remitted or who have experienced a recurrence.

Three main findings have emerged from this study. The first is that two-year remissions of the 24 symptoms studied were very common for those in both study groups. The median cumulative two-year remission rate was found to be 93% for borderline patients and 97% for Axis II comparison subjects. The cumulative rates of four-year remissions of many of the 24 symptoms studied were substantially lower than the cumulative rates of two-year remissions reported by both borderline patients and Axis II comparison subjects. More specifically, the median cumulative four-year remission rate was found to be 74% for borderline patients and 89% for Axis II comparison subjects.

The second main finding is that the rates of recurrence of the 24 symptoms being studied were quite high after a two-year remission but somewhat lower after a four-year remission. More specifically, the median cumulative recurrence rate for borderline patients was 75% after a two-year remission and 56% after a four-year remission. A similar pattern was found for Axis II comparison subjects—58% and 47%.

The third main finding is that acute symptoms had higher remission rates and lower recurrence rates than temperamental symptoms. This might be seen as a treatment effect, as all five of the comprehensive, empirically-based psychotherapies for BPD (Bateman & Fonagy, 1999; Clarkin, Levy, Lenzenweger, & Kernberg, 2007; Giesen-Bloo et al., 2006; Linehan, Armstrong, Suarez, Allmon, & Heard, 1991; McMain et al., 2009) are focused on acute symptoms. However, very few of the subjects in this study were ever in one of these treatments, because all of them are hard to access due to an insufficient number of trained practitioners. It may be that the supportive or eclectic therapies most patients reported being in also focused on these symptoms because of their association with turbulence in the therapeutic relationship, emergency room visits, and inpatient stays.

In contrast, 11 temperamental symptoms (all but dependency/masochism) were consistently found to have relatively low rates of remission and high rates of recurrence. Five of these symptoms are affective: chronic/major depression, chronic feelings of helplessness/hopelessness/worthlessness, chronic anger/frequent angry acts, chronic anxiety, and chronic loneliness/emptiness. The other temperamental symptoms showing this pattern of relatively low rates of remission and high rates of recurrence were odd thinking/unusual perceptual experiences, non-delusional paranoia, general impulsivity, intolerance of aloneness, abandonment/engulfment/annihilation concerns, and counterdependency/serious conflict over help/care. These symptoms, which span the cognitive, impulsive, and interpersonal sectors of borderline psychopathology, shared this pattern in a less severe and less consistent manner than found for affective symptoms. However, they, too, are among the more temperamental and less turbulent of the symptoms of BPD.

Taken together, these findings have important clinical implications. In general, they give clinicians a cognitive map of what to expect over time. They suggest patience on the part of clinicians and encouraging acceptance on the part of patients in dealing with the affective and other temperamental symptoms of BPD. They also suggest that the acute symptoms of BPD in general (not just self-harm and suicide attempts) are more responsive to treatment than previously recognized. However, it is not clear if treatment needs to focus on identifying the symptoms that are so troublesome, such as being manipulative and demanding, or if helping a patient take risks to have a more supportive set of relationships and a meaningful occupation are more helpful. In all likelihood, both approaches being applied concurrently would probably yield the best result.

The results of these studies provide proof that the symptoms of BPD are not chronic, but in many cases have high rates of remission. This is particularly so for the symptoms we have labeled "acute" symptoms. Most recently, we have found high rates of recurrence, particularly for the temperamental symptoms of BPD. This dichotomy will not surprise clinicians who know from experience that the dysphoria and dependency characteristic of many borderline patients are the most resistant to change. Whether this is related to a sub-threshold mood disorder, their basic temperament, or disappointment and shame at the life they are currently living, is unclear.

The CLPS study has published three papers related to changes in the *DSM-IV* symptoms of BPD over time. In the first of these studies, Shea and colleagues (2002) found that the number of BPD symptoms declined significantly over the first year of follow-up. The mean number of BPD criteria was about seven at baseline, about five at six-month follow-up, and about four at one-year follow-up.

McGlashan and associates (2005) studied the stability of the symptoms of BPD over two years. They found that the most prevalent and least changeable criteria for BPD were affective instability and anger. They also found that the least prevalent and most changeable criteria were self-injury and frantic efforts to avoid abandonment. They concluded that BPD and other personality disorders studied were hybrids of traits and symptomatic behaviors—which roughly correspond to our concept of temperamental and acute symptoms.

Gunderson and colleagues reported on the 10-year course of BPD (2011). In terms of criteria over time, they found that the mean number of criteria met for BPD decreased from about seven at baseline to about four in the first year, and thereafter steadily decreased at a rate of 0.29 criteria per year to a low of about 2 at 10 years. They also found that the rates of decline for each of the nine *DSM-IV* BPD criteria were similar, with those that were most prevalent at baseline remaining most prevalent after 10 years of prospective follow-up.

Clinical Vignette 1   DOMINANCE OF TEMPERAMENTAL SYMPTOMS OVER TIME

Ms. A was a single, 24-year-old female at entrance into the study. She was a high school graduate working at a "big box" store stocking shelves. Her father had died when she was a young child, and her mother struggled to support Ms. A and her two younger siblings.

Ms. A had a dramatic onset to her symptoms. After remembering long "forgotten" experiences of sexual abuse by two older male cousins, she became enraged, engaged in violent temper outbursts involving property destruction, and reported numerous quasi-psychotic symptoms. She also cut herself for the first time and made a non-lethal suicide attempt by overdosing on aspirin.

When initially assessed, she reported all of the 24 symptoms being studied except for substance abuse, promiscuity, treatment regressions, or countertransference problems. With added support and structure as well as non-aggressive pharmacotherapy, her acute symptoms of BPD resolved relatively rapidly and have not returned.

However, her some of her temperamental symptoms have remained relatively constant and have strongly interfered with her vocational performance and her maintenance of close friendships and establishment of romantic relationships. She is typically dysphoric in multiple ways, extremely worried about being abandoned, and is unusually dependent on her family and her therapist.

Eventually, her reluctance to face anxiety provoking situations led to her giving up her job and relying for support on disability payments. As her friends moved on with their lives, she has not replaced them and is basically alone in the world except for her family of origin and her treatment team.

While no longer meeting criteria for any disorder, and being in good physical health, she refuses to take the initiative to look for work or make a friend. She is aware of how limited her life is, but is dominated by her anxiety, abandonment concerns, and undue dependency. She also worries about what will happen to her when her mother dies but does not reach out to her for companionship or support. She occasionally complains of feelings of loneliness, but seems to prefer the life of a fearful loner to taking any risks or making any changes.

Clinical Vignette 2   INTERMITTENT ACUTE SYMPTOMS INTERFERE WITH QUALITY OF LIFE

Ms. B was a 27-year-old single woman at study entrance. She had had multiple prior hospitalizations. Most were for suicidal ideation or attempts. She began treatment during her index admission with a new psychiatrist who saw her for therapy and medication management.

Gradually, the interval between hospitalizations increased, and her suicidality decreased. She repeatedly tried to work, but ended up being fired. She also made friends easily, but none of these relationships was long lasting.

She gradually gave up her alcohol abuse and promiscuity, which had made her life chaotic and disorganized. In fact, her most persistent acute symptom was verbal outbursts. When frustrated, she would "speak her mind" at work and be fired for her "honesty." The same pattern was evident in her friendships. Her relationships were not really turbulent but rather tended to drift away after a verbal outburst or two.

She was aware of this pattern at work and in her relationships. However, her only enduring relationships were with her older sister and her therapist. Both would tolerate these episodic outbursts of self-righteousness without ending the relationship. In addition, she stopped working and was supported by Social Security disability benefits.

Over time, her anger lessened in intensity, and she had fewer outbursts as the consequences became increasingly painful for her. Yet her life has remained somewhat barren despite a good deal of activity on her part (e.g., joining a book club and then quitting it, taking dance lessons and then not having time to keep her appointments).

Ms. B and her therapist are working on this pattern and trying to understand if it is due to untreated attention deficit hyperactivity disorder (ADHD) or some type of residual general impulsivity. They are also considering whether it is due to some combination of the two. A trial of a stimulant has begun to assess its effects on her disorganization. They are also working on helping Ms. B keep her commitments so that she does not feel so ashamed of herself for going from one thing to another without finishing anything successfully.

Symptomatic Remissions and Recurrences of the Borderline Diagnosis

M any clinicians are reluctant to treat or actively avoid treating patients with BPD. This is so because of the interpersonal difficulties that tend to arise during such a treatment, such as serious treatment regressions and countertransference problems. It is also true that this aversion to treating those with BPD is partly due to the idea that BPD and, in fact, all personality disorders are chronic disorders. This belief, which was enshrined in the *DSM-III* description of personality disorders (American Psychiatric Association, 1980) has persisted despite the fact that there was extensive evidence from the longitudinal studies of Lee Robins (1966) and George Vaillant (1977) that those with personality disorders tend to get better or symptomatically remit as they grow older (and if they get the support and encouragement they need to mature and grow).

SYMPTOMATIC REMISSIONS

Patients with BPD met criteria for remission if they no longer met DIB-R and *DSM-III-R* criteria for BPD for a period of at least two years.

Comparison subjects met criteria for symptomatic remission if they no longer met criteria for their primary Axis II disorder for two or more years.

This definition does not mean that those with BPD (or another personality disorder) had no symptoms of their original diagnosis. Rather, residual symptoms were common, but the person would not typically be judged by an observer to still meet criteria for a personality disorder.

Table 7.1 summarizes the rates of remission experienced over the course of 16 years of prospective follow-up by those in both study groups. It should be noted that we assessed remission rates at six-year follow-up (Zanarini, Frankenburg, et al., 2003), 10-year follow-up (Zanarini, Frankenburg, Reich, & Fitzmaurice, 2010b), and 16-year follow-up (Zanarini et al., 2012).

As can be seen, three main findings concerning symptomatic remissions emerge from these studies. The first is that those in both study groups have

TABLE 7.1 CUMULATIVE RATES OF REMISSION FOR BORDERLINE PATIENTS AND AXIS II COMPARISON SUBJECTS OVER 16 YEARS OF PROSPECTIVE FOLLOW-UP

	2 YR FU	4 YR FU	6 YR FU	8 YR FU	10 YR FU	12 YR FU	14 YR FU	16 YR FU
			Remissions Lasting 2 Years					
BPD	35	55	76	88	91	95	97	99
OPD	88	96	99	99	99	99	99	99
			Remissions Lasting 4 Years					
BPD		29	47	67	80	84	90	95
OPD		86	94	95	97	97	97	97
			Remissions Lasting 6 Years					
BPD			28	44	63	78	82	90
OPD			86	94	95	97	97	97
			Remissions Lasting 8 Years					
BPD				28	43	57	70	78
OPD				85	94	95	97	97

higher remission rates the longer the time from their index admission. For borderline patients, 35% had a two-year remission by the time of the first wave of follow-up, while 99% of borderline patients had a two-year remission by the time of the latest completed wave of follow-up (i.e., 16 years after their index admission). In fact, the rate of remission for borderline patients slows over time, with 88% having had a remission by the time of the eight-year follow-up, and only an additional 11% having their first remission during the next eight years.

The second main finding is that the longer the length of remission for borderline patients, the lower the rates of remission. While 99% of borderline patients had a two-year remission, 95% had a four-year remission, 90% had a six-year remission, and 78% had an eight-year remission. This is not true for Axis II comparison subjects. The remission rates only declined from 99% for a two-year remission to 97% for an eight-year remission.

The third main finding is that borderline patients had a significantly slower time-to-remission than Axis II comparison subjects. Looked at another way, at least 85% of these comparison subjects had achieved a remission by the first time period possible.

It is also notable that these remissions were more stable than those achieved by borderline patients, as 99% had a two-year remission by the end of 16 years of prospective follow-up, while 97% had a four-year remission, a six-year remission, and an eight-year remission. This is so despite the fact that all of the people in the study were young adults with suicidal concerns and less than optimal support at the start of the study, proving the severity of borderline psychopathology initially and its persistence over time relative to other forms of personality disorder.

SYMPTOMATIC RECURRENCES

Symptomatic recurrences are the flip side of the stability or relative lack thereof of symptomatic remissions. Table 7.2 summarizes the rates of recurrence experienced over the course of 16 years of prospective follow-up by those in both study groups. It should be noted that recurrences are

TABLE 7.2 CUMULATIVE RATES OF RECURRENCE FOR BORDERLINE
PATIENTS AND AXIS II COMPARISON SUBJECTS OVER 16 YEARS
OF PROSPECTIVE FOLLOW-UP

	2 Yrs After 1st Remission	4 Yrs After 1st Remission	6 Yrs After 1st Remission	8 Yrs After 1st Remission	10 Yrs After 1st Remission	12 Yrs After 1st Remission	14 Yrs After 1st Remission
	Recurrence After Remissions Lasting 2 Years						
BPD	16	21	30	33	34	36	36
OPD	3	3	3	5	5	7	7
	Recurrence After Remissions Lasting 4 Years						
BPD	7	16	21	22	25	25	
OPD	0	0	2	2	4	4	
	Recurrence After Remissions Lasting 6 Years						
BPD	10	15	16	19	19		
OPD	0	2	2	4	4		
	Recurrence After Remissions Lasting 8 Years						
BPD	5	7	10	10			
OPD	2	2	4	4			

assessed by the number of years that have elapsed since the first remission, and not at particular time periods as remissions are assessed.

Three main findings concerning symptomatic recurrences emerge from these studies. The first is that those in both study groups had higher recurrence rates the shorter the time of first remission. For borderline patients, 36% had a symptomatic recurrence after a two-year remission, 25% had a recurrence after a four-year remission, 19% had a recurrence after a six-year remission, and 10% had a recurrence after an eight-year remission. For Axis II comparison subjects, 7% had a recurrence after a two-year remission, and 4% had a recurrence after a four-, six-, and eight-year remission.

The second main finding is that the greater the number of years after first remission, the higher the rate of recurrence. For borderline patients, the rate of recurrence two years after a two-year remission was 16%, and the rate after 14 years was 36%. The rates for Axis II comparison subjects did not increase as much with time (3% vs. 7%).

The third main finding is that borderline patients had a significantly faster time-to-recurrence than Axis II comparison subjects for recurrences following two-, four-, and six-year remissions. However, no difference was found in time-to-recurrence after an eight-year remission.

The CLPS study found similar rates of remission for BPD at 10-year follow-up (Gunderson, Stout, et al., 2011). More specifically, 85% of *DSM-IV* borderline subjects no longer met criteria for BPD for 12 months after 10 years of prospective follow-up (as opposed to 88% in the MSAD study having a symptomatic remission of at least two years after eight years of prospective follow-up). After a 12-month remission, however, only 12% experienced a symptomatic recurrence of BPD (as opposed to 36% of the borderline subjects in the MSAD study having a symptomatic recurrence after a two-year remission).

These findings concerning borderline psychopathology have given hope to patients, their families, and the mental health professionals treating them. These results also challenged the prevailing view that BPD is a "chronic" disorder with a poor prognosis. In fact, these results seemed to suggest that BPD, even for former inpatients suffering from severe borderline psychopathology, is a diagnosis with a good symptomatic prognosis; a prognosis in which substantial symptomatic improvement is to be expected for most patients.

Despite these findings, many clinicians still believe that BPD is a chronic disorder with little hope of improvement over time. Taken together, these results suggest that the course of BPD is very different than that of mood disorders. While major depression (Mueller et al., 1999; Solomon et al., 1997) and bipolar disorder (Coryell et al., 1995; Tohen et al., 2000) are relatively quick to remit, recurrences are common. In contrast, BPD is relatively slow to remit, but recurrences are relatively rare. Looked at another way, our findings suggest that BPD is relatively stable over time compared to mood disorders, for example, but mutable over more sustained periods of time.

Despite the reluctance of many mental health professionals to accept that BPD is a "good prognosis" diagnosis, it is key that patients and their family members learn that symptomatic improvement can be expected. There are a number of groups that have developed training programs for the family members of those with BPD. Chief among them is the National Educational Alliance for Borderline Personality Disorder (NEA-BPD), which has developed a peer training program for family members interested in helping their relative with BPD. This program, Family Connections, provides family members with information about BPD and teaches some of Linehan's Dialectical Behavioral Therapy (DBT) skills (Linehan et al., 1991), which enable family members to be more effective and less stressed as they relate to their relative with BPD (Hoffman, Fruzzetti, & Buteau, 2007).

Patients with BPD also need to know the latest information about BPD. In order to provide that information, our group has developed an internet-based psychoeducation program for early treatment for BPD—BPDPSYCHOED—which has proven to be clinically useful in decreasing symptom severity and improving psychosocial functioning for periods up to one year (Zanarini, Conkey, Temes, & Fitzmaurice, 2017).

8

Prevalence and Predictors of Physically Self-Destructive Acts over Time

Self-mutilation and help-seeking suicide attempts are among the few almost pathognomonic symptoms of BPD (Zanarini, Gunderson, Frankenburg, & Chauncey, 1990). They are both among the acute symptoms of BPD—having a pattern of relatively rapid remission, being among the best markers for the disorder, and often the reason for costly forms of psychiatric care, such as hospitalizations or day programs.

This chapter explores the prevalence of self-mutilation, suicide threats, and suicide attempts. It also explores the predictors of these three separate forms of physically self-destructive acts.

PREDICTORS OF SELF-MUTILATION OVER 10 YEARS OF PROSPECTIVE FOLLOW-UP

Eleven variables were found to be significant predictors of an episode of self-harm at any follow-up period (Zanarini, Laudate, Frankenburg,

---

Box 8.1   SIGNIFICANT BIVARIATE PREDICTORS OF SELF-MUTILATION OVER 10 YEARS OF PROSPECTIVE FOLLOW-UP

Female gender

Severity of dysphoric affects[1]

Severity of dysphoric cognitions[1]

Severity of dissociation[1]

Major depression[1]

Childhood history of sexual abuse

Severity of childhood history of other abuse

Severity of childhood history of neglect

Adult sexual assault[1]

Adult physical assault[1]

Lifetime number of episodes of self-mutilation at baseline

[1] Time-varying predictors of self-mutilation. The other five were assessed once at baseline.

Reich, & Fitzmaurice, 2011). These 11 variables, some of which were baseline variables and some of which were time-varying variables, are shown in Box 8.1.

Six of these variables were found to significantly predict self-mutilation in joint analyses. They are shown in Box 8.2.

It is not surprising that being female is a predictor of episodes of self-mutilation, as it has previously been found that self-harm is more common over time among women than men with BPD (Zanarini, Frankenburg, Hennen, et al., 2003). It is a new finding that the severity of overvalued ideas of being bad heightens the risk of self-mutilation over time. This finding suggests that firmly held negative beliefs about the self, which might be intensified by either interpersonal disappointments or concurrent major depressive episodes, are an important predictor of the likelihood that a borderline patient will engage in self-mutilation over time.

Box 8.2 **SIGNIFICANT MULTIVARIATE PREDICTORS OF SELF-MUTILATION OVER 10 YEARS OF PROSPECTIVE FOLLOW-UP**

Female gender
Severity of dysphoric cognitions[1]
Severity of dissociation[1]
Major depression[1]
Childhood history of sexual abuse
Adult sexual assault[1]

[1] Time-varying predictors of self-mutilation. The other two were assessed once at baseline.

Dissociation has long been associated with the borderline diagnosis. At times, it is seen as a core symptom of BPD (Zanarini, Gunderson, & Frankenburg, 1990) with a strong heritable component (Jang, Paris, Zweig-Frank, & Livesley, 1998). At other times, it is seen as a way of coping with the stress inherent in childhood sexual abuse or adult sexual assault (Herman & van der Kolk, 1987). Regardless of its etiology, it seems that being disengaged from one's feelings heightens the risk that a person with BPD will engage in self-mutilation at some point over a decade of prospective follow-up.

Our final multivariate predictors of self-mutilation over time are childhood sexual abuse and adult sexual assault. These findings, while important, need to be placed in context. More specifically, these factors are associated with a heightened risk of self-mutilation over time. These results do not mean that all borderline patients who mutilated themselves over time had a history of childhood sexual abuse, adult sexual assault, or both. Nor do they mean that all borderline patients who reported childhood and/or adult sexual abuse or assault deliberately hurt themselves physically over the course of the study.

However, five significant bivariate predictors were not significant in our multivariate model: severity of dysphoric affects, severity of other forms of childhood abuse, severity of childhood neglect, adult experiences of being physically assaulted by a partner or spouse, and lifetime number of episodes of self-mutilation at study entry. At first glance, it seems surprising that dysphoric affects would not be a significant multivariate risk factor for episodes of self-mutilation. But our results seem to suggest that painful overvalued ideas and the numbing effects of dissociation are substantially stronger risk factors than dysphoric affects, perhaps because they are more stable inner states than affects, which tend to be more reactive in nature. In addition, the presence of one or more episodes of major depression in a follow-up period may have subsumed some of the predictive power of our continuous measure of affective dysphoria.

It also seems surprising that the severity of non-sexual forms of childhood abuse and the severity of childhood neglect are not significant multivariate predictors of self-mutilation over time. This is particularly so because we had previously found a cross-sectional relationship between these variables in this study (Zanarini, Yong, et al., 2002). However, it may be that the effects of other forms of childhood abuse and childhood neglect attenuate over time, or at least their effects may attenuate more over time than the effects of childhood sexual abuse.

The lack of a significant multivariate relationship between adult experiences of physical abuse and self-mutilation over time does not seem particularly surprising. This is so partly because no cross-sectional study has found a significant link between childhood physical abuse and a history of self-mutilation (Zanarini, Yong, et al., 2002). This is also so because these abandonment-sensitive patients may interpret the actions of physically abusive partners or spouses as a sign of intense involvement that mitigates the need for the indirect communication inherent in self-mutilation (Hooley & Hoffman, 1999).

Finally, the lifetime number of episodes of self-mutilation reported at baseline failed to be a significant multivariate predictor of self-mutilation over time for borderline patients. The reasons for this are not clear. It may be that predictors closer in time to episodes of self-mutilation during the decade of prospective follow-up (i.e., time-varying predictors such as major depressive episodes) are stronger predictors of ongoing self-mutilation. It may also be that the pattern of self-mutilation engaged in prior to index admission was already waning for some patients.

REASONS FOR SELF-MUTILATION OVER 16 YEARS OF PROSPECTIVE FOLLOW-UP

We have also studied the reasons for self-harm for borderline patients with a more extensive history of self-harm at baseline (N = 133) and those with a less extensive history of self-harm during their index admission (N = 129) (Zanarini, Laudate, Frankenburg, Wedig, & Fitzmaurice, 2013). All told, 262 borderline patients, or 90%, had a lifetime history of self-harm at study entry. We studied seven reasons for self-harm over 16 years of prospective follow-up. Two were interpersonal: feeling angry or frustrated with someone and to get attention. Two others were inner states of an affective nature: to relieve anxiety and to control emotional pain. Three others were internally directed reasons of a cognitive nature: feeling numb or dead (depersonalization), to punish oneself, or to prevent being hurt in a worse way. These groups were not significantly different from one another on either of the interpersonally directed reasons for self-mutilation studied. However, those in the more extensive group were significantly more likely to report each of the five internally-directed reasons studied. The results of this study suggest that border-line patients with a more extensive history of self-mutilation are best distinguished from those with a less extensive history by episodes of self-harm that are motivated, at least in part, by dysphoric inner states.

These findings, when taken together, have important clinical implications. Clinicians may overestimate the importance of the interpersonal reasons for self-harm. Or looked at another way, they may not be mindful of the ways that borderline patients are using self-injury to try to soothe themselves, punish themselves, or prevent further punishment or harm. Awareness of this inner-directed set of reasons may lead to more empathic or validating responses to the threat of self-harm or actual episodes of self-mutilation. It may also help clinicians to encourage their borderline patients to be more curious and more forthright about their motivations for self-harm.

PREDICTORS OF SUICIDE THREATS OVER 16 YEARS OF PROSPECTIVE FOLLOW-UP

Suicide threats are often engaged in by borderline patients as well (Wedig, Frankenburg, Reich, Fitzmaurice, & Zanarini, 2013). More specifically, the following prevalence rates for suicide threats were found at the study's nine two-year-long measurement periods: 57.6% at baseline, 38.5% at two-year follow-up, 26.0% at four-year follow-up, 17.4% at six-year follow-up, 16.1% at eight-year follow-up, 12.9% at 10-year follow-up, 12.7% at 12-year follow-up, 10.5% at 14-year follow-up, and 10.8% at 16-year follow-up.

Nineteen time-varying predictors of prevalence over time were studied: 14 of these predictors reflected inner affective and cognitive states (percentage of time experienced—0–100% of the time), and five reflected interpersonal behaviors (presence/absence). (Each of these time-varying variables predicted suicide threats occurring in the same time period as the predictor occurred. For example, feeling abandoned during the two years from two- to four-year follow-up was studied as a predictor of suicide threats during the same two-year period.)

Table 8.1 lists these predictors. All of these predictors were significant in bivariate analyses (i.e., each significantly predicted a suicide threat at that time point).

However, only four of these predictors were significant in multivariate analyses (where all bivariate predictors are tested for significance at the same time). These predictors are: feeling abandoned and hopeless, and being demanding and manipulative (Box 8.3).

The results of this study suggest that suicide threats are often related to emotions (but not cognitions) connected with interpersonal relationships. Suicide threats may function, albeit maladaptively, to regulate these emotions that are aroused by interpersonal relationships that may seem

TABLE 8.1 BIVARIATE TIME-VARYING PREDICTORS OF SUICIDE THREATS OVER 16 YEARS OF PROSPECTIVE FOLLOW-UP

Severity of Affective States	Severity of Cognitive States	Interpersonal Symptoms (presence/absence)
Abandoned	Completely out of control	Devaluation
All alone	Like no one cares about me	Manipulation
Desperate	Like people hate me	Sadism
Furious or enraged inside	Like the pain will never end	Demandingness
Hopeless	Misunderstood	Entitlement
Hurt		
In agony		
Overwhelmed		
Very angry inside		

in jeopardy of failing, or are failing. It should be noted that the prevalence rates reported may be an underestimate, as it is often difficult for some people to differentiate between a threat and just telling someone about feeling suicidal with no intention to act.

Suicide threats also seem related to outmoded survival strategies: being manipulative and being demanding. This is not surprising, but it differs from the most salient predictors of self-mutilation. This may because self-mutilation is often conducted in private and may be kept secret. However,

Box 8.3 **MULTIVARIATE TIME-VARYING PREDICTORS OF SUICIDE THREATS OVER 16 YEARS OF PROSPECTIVE FOLLOW-UP**

Severity of feeling abandoned
Severity of feeling hopeless
Being manipulative
Being demanding

suicide threats are by their very nature interpersonal, as are being manipulative and demanding.

PREDICTORS OF SUICIDE ATTEMPTS OVER 16
YEARS OF PROSPECTIVE FOLLOW-UP

Finally, we studied predictors of actual suicide attempts over time (Wedig
et al., 2012). Nineteen variables were found to be significant bivariate
predictors of suicide attempts (Box 8.4).

Eight of these, seven of which were time-varying, remained significant
in multivariate analyses (Box 8.5).

Three of these predictors are co-occurring disorders—major depression, substance abuse, and PTSD—all of which could increase the desperation and/or impulsivity of borderline patients. Three other predictors are
symptoms of BPD: presence of self-harm, affective instability, and more
severe dissociation. These predictors also could increase the dysphoria
and/or the action orientation of borderline patients. There was one predictor related to family history of psychiatric disorder: having had a close
relative commit suicide. Once the taboo of committing suicide is breached
within a family, clinical experience suggests that it increases the odds of
another family member's attempting suicide. It may be that suicide seems
normative in these families. It may also be that family members suffer
from the same constellation of symptoms and/or personality traits that
predispose one to attempt suicide. Finally, adult sexual assault could also
be associated with a suicide attempt as it would engender deep feelings of
rage, powerlessness, and shame.

RATES OF COMPLETED SUICIDE

Over 16 years of prospective follow-up, 13 borderline patients and one
Axis II comparison subject committed suicide. An additional borderline
patient committed suicide after 20 years of prospective follow-up. Thus,

---

Box 8.4 SIGNIFICANT BIVARIATE PREDICTORS OF SUICIDE ATTEMPTS OVER 16 YEARS OF PROSPECTIVE FOLLOW-UP

Age

Major Depressive Disorder[1]

Substance Use Disorder[1]

PTSD[1]

Presence of Self-Harm[1]

Severity of Dissociative Experiences[1]

Number of Baseline Suicide Attempts

Number of Baseline Psychiatric Hospitalizations

Baseline GAF

Severity of Childhood Neglect

Childhood Sexual Abuse

Adult Sexual Assault[1]

Adult Physical Assault[1]

On Social Security Disability Income [1]

Caretaker Suicide Completion

Affective Instability[1]

Impulsivity[1]

Higher Neuroticism[1]

Lower Extraversion[1]

[1] Time-varying predictors of suicide attempts. The other seven were assessed once at baseline.

---

our rate of completed suicide is either 4.5% or 4.8%, depending on the waves of follow-up considered. In either case, it is substantially lower than the 9–10% found in two of the three long-term follow-back studies that assessed this outcome (Paris et al., 1987; Stone, 1990). It may be that our rate was substantially lower because of the more supportive treatments that our patients received. It may also have been lower because of the

---

**Box 8.5   SIGNIFICANT MULTIVARIATE PREDICTORS
OF SUICIDE ATTEMPTS OVER 16 YEARS
OF PROSPECTIVE FOLLOW-UP**

Major Depressive Disorder[1]

Substance Use Disorder[1]

PTSD[1]

Presence of Self-harm[1]

Severity of Dissociative Experiences[1]

Adult Sexual Assault[1]

Caretaker Suicide Completion

Affective Instability[1]

[1] Time-varying predictors of suicide attempts. The other one was assessed once at baseline.

---

greater awareness in therapy of childhood adversities than in these older
studies conducted in the 1980s.

OTHER DEATHS

Over 16 years of prospective follow-up, 13 borderline patients (4.5%) and
one Axis II comparison subject (1.4%) died of natural causes. Five additional borderline patients (1.7%) died of natural causes during the following two waves of follow-up (18- and 20-year follow-ups). Thus, 6.2%
of borderline patients and 1.4% of Axis II comparison subjects died of
natural causes after 20 years of prospective follow-up.

Overall, 11% of borderline patients and 2.8% of Axis II comparison
subjects died of all causes put together over 20 years of prospective follow-
up. While a few people died of serious illnesses not strongly related to
lifestyle choices (e.g., breast cancer), most borderline patients who died
of natural causes died of weight- and/or smoking-related illnesses. And it
is important to note that, on average, the subjects in this study were only

about 47 years old at this point in time. These findings strongly suggest that all mental health clinicians and primary care physicians need to pay focused attention to the physical health of their patients with BPD. This is so because many of these natural deaths were more than 20–30 years premature compared to figures obtained from community samples (Kochanek, Murphy, Xu, & Tejada-Vera, 2016). This is a totally new finding, but one that is particularly unfortunate and one that we hope will serve as a wakeup call for all health professionals treating these vulnerable patients.

9

Additional Symptom Areas over Time

This chapter is a discussion of findings pertaining to symptom areas common among those with BPD but that are not part of *DSM-IV/-5* or do not have the importance that our results suggest they deserve.

AFFECTS OVER TIME

This section is devoted to affects that are common among those with BPD and the source of serious suffering but are not part of our official nomenclature.

Anxiety over Time

We assessed five anxiety symptoms reported by borderline patients and Axis II comparison subjects over 16 years of prospective follow-up

(Zanarini, Frankenburg, & Fitzmaurice, 2014). These symptoms were: anxious, scared, terrified, completely panicked, and an aggregate of the four—any anxiety. Each variable reflected the percentage of time that that type of anxiety was experienced at each study period (e.g., 10% of the time, 40% of the time). The mean score for any anxiety among patients with BPD was 41.4 at baseline and 18.3 at 16-year follow-up. In comparison, the mean score for any anxiety among Axis II comparison subjects was 24.5 at baseline and 10.3 at 16-year follow-up (Figure 9.1).

It was found that each symptom and our composite score for overall anxiety was about twice as severe among borderline patients as among Axis II comparison subjects. In addition, borderline patients reported feeling anxious 38% less of the time over the years of follow-up, scared 70% less of the time, terrified 74% less of the time, and completely panicked 60% less of the time. And the percentage of time they reported overall anxiety decreased by 58%. Among borderline patients, two variables were found to be significant multivariate predictors of severity of overall anxiety: severity of non-sexual childhood abuse and higher trait neuroticism.

The results of this study suggest that anxiety symptoms form a distinct profile for borderline patients—a profile related to both childhood adversity of an emotional, verbal, and/or physical nature, and a vulnerable temperament high in neuroticism. These findings have clinical implications. First, they point to the subjective suffering of borderline patients caused

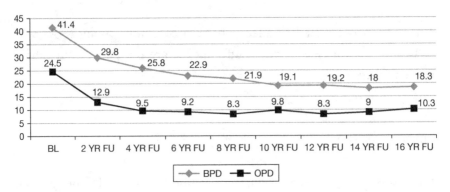

Figure 9.1 Percentage of time borderline patients and Axis II comparison subjects reported feeling anxious.

by these high levels of anxiety. Second, our group (Zanarini, Frankenburg, Reich, & Fitzmaurice, 2010a) and the CLPS group (Skodol et al., 2002) have noted that a sizeable minority of borderline patients cannot function well vocationally, particularly on a full-time basis. Clinical experience suggests that high levels of anxiety and the wish to avoid feeling even more anxious are associated with avoidance of obtaining and keeping full-time work or being enrolled as a full-time student.

SHAME OVER TIME

We also assessed the percentage of time borderline patients and Axis II comparison subjects reported feelings of shame over 16 years of prospective follow-up (Karan, Niesten, Frankenburg, Fitzmaurice, & Zanarini, 2014). The mean score for shame among patients with BPD was 50.7 at baseline and 17.8 at 16-year follow-up (i.e., borderline patients reported feeling shame 51% of the time at baseline and 18% of the time at 16-year follow-up). In comparison, the mean score for shame among Axis II comparison subjects was 27.0 at baseline and 8.6 at 16-year follow-up (Figure 9.2).

Borderline patients reported significantly higher levels (2.6 times) of shame across 16 years of follow-up than did Axis II comparison subjects.

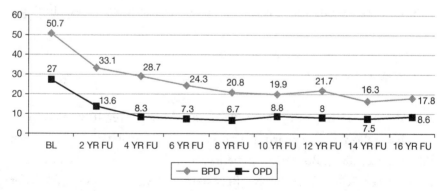

Figure 9.2 Percentage of time borderline patients and Axis II comparison subjects reported feeling shame.

However, the severity of shame decreased significantly over time for those in both groups (78%). Regarding risk factors, four lifetime adversity risk factors were found to be significantly associated with feelings of shame: severity of childhood sexual abuse, severity of other forms of childhood abuse, severity of childhood neglect (which was mostly emotional in nature), and severity of adult abuse or adversity (including physical assault and rape). Two of these factors (severity of childhood sexual abuse and severity of childhood neglect) remained significant in multivariate analyses. Taken together, the results of this study suggest that borderline patients struggle with intense but decreasing feelings of shame. They also suggest that childhood adversities are significant risk factors for this dysphoric affective state.

Clinically, this state is very important and impedes progress for those with BPD, as it is an inner state that borderline patients experience with even the slightest interpersonal disappointment or most inadvertent interpersonal slight. As a result of this reactive quality to shame, it is often difficult for those with BPD to enter close relationships for fear of being shamed, or to enjoy the competitive aspects of work for fear of failure and the resulting feelings of shame.

COGNITIONS OVER TIME

Below we discuss this often overlooked area of borderline psychopathology.

Dissociation over Time

In addition, we studied the severity of dissociation over 10 years of prospective follow-up (Zanarini, Frankenburg, Jager-Hyman, Reich, & Fitzmaurice, 2008). Borderline patients reported a mean total Dissociative Experiences Scale (DES) score (Bernstein & Putnam, 1986) of 21.8 at baseline (and Axis II comparison subjects reported a mean score of 7.5). By the time of their 10-year follow-up, the mean total DES score reported by borderline patients had declined to 8.5 (and that of Axis II comparison subjects had declined to 3.9) (Figure 9.3).

The mean total DES score reported by borderline patients at baseline is approximately two and a half times larger than the corresponding mean for Axis II comparison subjects. The relative change from baseline to 10-year follow-up resulted in an approximately 43% decline for Axis II comparison subjects. In contrast, the relative decline from baseline to 10-year follow-up is approximately 61% for borderline patients.

As for the three sub-scale scores of the DES, the relative differences of 2.44, 3.36, and 2.54 for diagnosis indicate that the mean absorption (basically normal forms of dissociation, such as driving home and not remembering the details of the trip home), depersonalization, and amnesia scores reported by borderline patients at baseline were approximately 2.5, 3, and 2.5 times larger, respectively, than the corresponding means for Axis II comparison subjects. The relative change from baseline to 10-year follow-up resulted in approximately 55%, 26%, and 32% declines among Axis II comparison subjects for absorption, depersonalization, and amnesia, respectively. In contrast, the relative decline from baseline to 10-year follow-up is approximately 65% (absorption), 59% (depersonalization), and 62% (amnesia) for borderline patients.

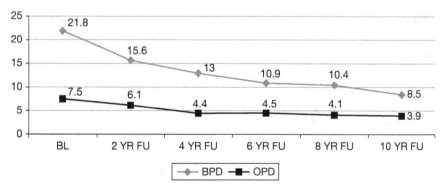

Figure 9.3 Percentage of time borderline patients and Axis II comparison subjects reported feeling dissociated.

We also examined the mean total DES scores of three sub-groups of borderline patients defined by their baseline mean total DES score: high (26%), moderate (42%), and low or normal (32%) (Figure 9.4).

Those in the high and moderate baseline DES groups had a significantly faster rate of decline than those in the low DES group. It was also found that those in the high DES group had a significantly faster rate of decline than those in the moderate group. However, those in all three groups experienced a significant decline in mean total DES score from baseline to 10-year follow-up (with relative decline of 73% in the high group, 66% in the moderate group, and 38% in the low group).

We also studied remissions and recurrences of those in the high baseline DES score group (i.e., score of 30 or higher, indicative of a trauma-spectrum disorder). Over 90% of borderline patients reporting very high levels of dissociation at baseline experienced a remission of this high level of dissociation over time. However, slightly more than a third of borderline patients who experienced a remission later experienced a recurrence of severe dissociative symptoms. As for the borderline patients who had a mean DES score in the low or moderate range at baseline, about 8% experienced a new onset of severe dissociative symptoms over the 10 years of prospective follow-up. (These analyses were limited to borderline patients, as only two [2.8%] of Axis II comparison subjects had mean DES scores

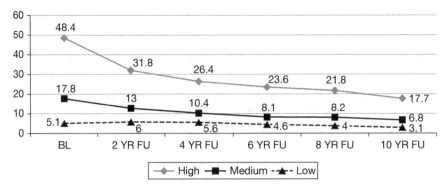

Figure 9.4 Percentage of time baseline severity groups of borderline patients reported feeling dissociated.

of 30 or more at baseline; both had a remission, neither had a recurrence, and only one additional comparison subject had a new onset.) These results suggest that the severity of dissociation declines significantly over time for even severely ill borderline patients. However, it remains a recurring problem for over a third of those with DES scores that initially were in the range associated with trauma-spectrum disorders.

SEVENTEEN SPECIFIC COGNITIONS ASSESSED BY THE DIB-R OVER 16 YEARS OF PROSPECTIVE FOLLOW-UP

Each of the five main types of thought studied (odd thinking, unusual perceptual experiences, non-delusional paranoia, quasi-psychotic thought, and true-psychotic thought) was reported by a significantly higher percentage of borderline patients than Axis II comparison subjects over time (Zanarini, Frankenburg, Wedig, & Fitzmaurice, 2013). Each of these types of thought, except true-psychotic thought, declined significantly over time for those in both groups. Eleven of the 17 more specific forms of thought studied were also reported by a significantly higher percentage of borderline patients over the years of follow-up: magical thinking, overvalued ideas, recurrent illusions, depersonalization, derealization, undue suspiciousness, ideas of reference, other paranoid ideation, quasi-psychotic delusions, quasi-psychotic hallucinations, and true-psychotic hallucinations. Fourteen specific forms of thought were found to decline significantly over time for those in both groups: all forms of thought just mentioned, except true-psychotic hallucinations, plus marked superstitiousness, sixth sense, telepathy, and clairvoyance. These results suggest that disturbed cognitions are common among borderline patients and distinguishing for the disorder. They also suggest that these symptoms decline substantially over time but remain a problem, particularly those of a nonpsychotic nature.

COGNITIVE SYMPTOMS OF BPD AND THE *DSM* NOMENCLATURE

Neither *DSM-III* nor *DSM-III-R* had a cognitive criterion for BPD. One was added in *DSM-IV*: "transient, stress-related paranoid ideation or severe dissociative symptoms." Clearly, the cognitive symptoms of borderline patients are more complex than this one criterion conveys. It is also clear from clinical experience that the paranoia and dissociation of BPD get worse with stress but are often present in a latent fashion over sustained periods of time. In addition, it is clear that only a minority of those with BPD ever have high levels of dissociation, but moderate levels are more common. Yet the proposed dimensional approach to BPD in *DSM-5* does not list even one cognitive symptom (American Psychiatric Association, 2013). Instead, all the cognitive symptoms we found in our borderline patients were assigned to the criteria set for schizotypal personality disorder. It is difficult to understand this choice, as it seems to be following a theory of personality rather than the clinical reality presented by those with BPD. And in this regard, it is important to remember that less than 7% of the borderline patients in this study met *DSM-III-R* criteria for schizotypal personality disorder (Zanarini et al., 1998a).

10

Psychosocial Functioning
over Time

P sychosocial functioning is a complex topic that involves various aspects of social and vocational functioning. It is also an area that is of great importance to those with BPD, their families, and the mental health professionals treating them.

PSYCHOSOCIAL FUNCTIONING OVER THE FIRST SIX YEARS OF PROSPECTIVE FOLLOW-UP

At six-year follow-up, the social and vocational functioning of 202 remitted borderline patients and 88 non-remitted borderline patients was compared (Zanarini, Frankenburg, Hennen, et al., 2005). ("Remission," as noted elsewhere, was defined as no longer meeting study criteria for BPD at one or more follow-up periods.) It was found that ever-remitted borderline patients had significantly better psychosocial functioning than never-remitted borderline patients on six of the 12 variables studied. More specifically, they were significantly more likely to have a good relationship with a spouse/partner and at least one parent; good work/school performance; a sustained work/school history, which was defined as consistently working or going to school for at least 50% of each study period; a GAF score of 61 or higher; and to have good overall psychosocial functioning, which was defined as having at least one emotionally sustaining relationship and a successful work/school record. (A "good or emotionally sustaining" relationship was defined as one that involved at least weekly contact and was judged by the patient to be close, without elements of either abuse or neglect. A "successful" vocational record was defined as both performing well at work or school and being able to do so in a sustained manner.)

It is clear that the symptomatic status of borderline patients seems to have a strong impact on their psychosocial functioning. While the social and vocational functioning of ever-remitted borderline patients improved steadily over time, that of never-remitted borderline patients was relatively steady in most areas. By the time of the six-year follow-up assessment, over a third of the remitted borderline patients were married or living with a partner, while only 14% of the never-remitted borderline patients were living in an intimate relationship. However, about a quarter of both ever-remitted and never-remitted borderline patients had children. Almost two-thirds of ever-remitted borderline patients, but less than half of never-remitted borderline patients, had an emotionally supportive relationship with a spouse or partner. Over three-quarters of ever-remitted borderline patients, but only about 60% of never-remitted borderline patients, had emotionally sustaining relationships with friends and at least one of their parents.

In the vocational realm, over three-quarters of ever-remitted borderline patients, but less than half of never-remitted borderline patients, had performed well at work or school, and were able to work or go to school in a sustained manner. In addition, over 40% of ever-remitted borderline patients had a professional, managerial, or technical occupation, but almost the same percentage were supported, at least in part, through governmental disability payments—many remaining on disability because of needing the attendant health insurance for their psychiatric treatment. In contrast, only 13% of never-remitted borderline patients had a high-level occupation, but about 75% were receiving disability payments. Over 80% of those in both groups used their leisure time in a meaningful manner, suggesting an area of strength for both types of borderline patients.

In terms of overall functioning, over 40% of ever-remitted borderline patients had a GAF in the good range, and over 65% had attained or maintained good overall psychosocial functioning. In contrast, no non-remitted borderline patient had a good GAF at six-year follow-up, and only about a quarter had attained or maintained good psychosocial functioning.

The reasons for these differences between ever-remitted and never-remitted borderline patients are unclear. It may be that the greater severity of BPD symptoms among the never-remitted borderline patients seriously impeded their psychosocial functioning. Alternatively, it may be that never-remitted and ever-remitted borderline patients may be different in other ways as well, such as having different temperaments, different childhood experiences, or some combination of the two. In any case, it is important to note that the psychosocial functioning of remitted patients continued to improve as time progressed, suggesting that they were somewhat belatedly achieving the milestones of young adulthood and not simply returning to a prodromal level of functioning. In addition, it is important to note that the pattern of steady, multifaceted improvement found in the current study has not been found for other serious psychiatric disorders, such as bipolar I disorder (Tohen et al., 2000).

We also compared borderline patients to Axis II comparison subjects. We found that borderline patients made overall psychosocial progress over time, as represented by a GAF score of 61 or higher or achieving criteria for good psychosocial functioning. However, this overall progress was achieved by a significantly lower percentage of borderline patients than by Axis II comparison subjects.

In terms of GAF scores, no borderline patient had a GAF score in the good range at baseline, but this figure increased to 33% by the time of the six-year follow-up. In a like manner, no Axis II comparison subject had a GAF score in the good range at baseline. However, by the time of the six-year follow-up, this figure had increased to 64%—almost double the rate found for borderline patients. The picture is much the same for the variable of good overall psychosocial functioning, which, unlike the GAF, does not assess an admixture of symptoms and psychosocial impairment (see Figure 10.1). The percentage of borderline patients judged to have good functioning in the social and vocational realms increased over the course of the study from 26% to 56%, while the percentage of Axis II comparison subjects increased from 58% to 73%—suggesting that Axis II comparison subjects were substantially less impaired psychosocially at baseline and at six-year follow-up than borderline patients were.

In terms of specific realms of functioning, borderline patients and Axis II comparison subjects functioned about the same in terms of being in a committed relationship, having children, and having emotionally sustaining relationships with others. The meaningful use of their leisure time was also about the same. However, there were significant differences found in the vocational realm. Borderline patients were significantly less

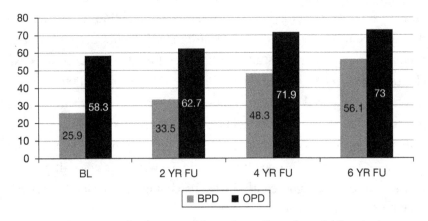

Figure 10.1 Percentage of each group with good overall psychosocial functioning.

able to perform at work or school than Axis II comparison subjects. They were also significantly less able to work or go to school in a sustained manner. In addition, they were about three times more likely to be receiving disability payments.

These results suggest that psychosocial improvement is both common among borderline patients and strongly related to their symptomatic status. They also suggest that those with BPD, particularly those who have never remitted by the time of the six-year follow-up, are more impaired in the vocational than in the social realm.

A NOTE OF CAUTION

These optimistic findings gave hope to borderline patients and their families that they could be expected to make psychosocial progress, particularly if they remitted from BPD. However, findings from three studies that encompassed the first 10 years and 16 years of psychosocial functioning suggested that these six-year findings might be too optimistic, and in fact, the psychosocial outlook for many with BPD was more guarded than previously recognized.

PSYCHOSOCIAL FUNCTIONING OVER FIRST 10 YEARS OF PROSPECTIVE FOLLOW-UP

In the first of these studies (Zanarini, Jacoby, Frankenburg, Reich, & Fitzmaurice, 2009), it was found that borderline patients were three times more likely to be receiving Social Security Disability Income (SSDI) benefits than were Axis II comparison subjects over time, although the prevalence rate for both groups remained relatively stable (roughly 40% vs. 15%). Forty percent of borderline patients on such payments at baseline were able to get off disability, but 43% of these patients subsequently went back on SSDI. Additionally, 39% of borderline patients who were not on disability at baseline started to receive federal benefits for the first time.

However, borderline patients on SSDI were not without psychosocial strengths. By the time of the 10-year follow-up, 55% had worked or gone to school at least 50% of the last two years, about 70% had a supportive relationship with at least one friend, and over 50% had a good relationship with a romantic partner. But those with BPD who had never been on disability were significantly more likely to achieve these outcomes over time.

These findings suggest that about half of borderline patients receiving federal disability benefits have some capacity to function vocationally. They also suggest that the social functioning of borderline patients on disability is better than their vocational functioning. However, it seems that intimate relationships with partners are harder to develop and maintain than relationships with friends.

It should also be noted that borderline patients who were never on disability benefits functioned substantially better in all areas. About 85% had a sustained vocational performance and a good relationship with at least one friend by the time of the ninth and tenth years of follow-up. In addition, almost 70% had an emotionally sustaining relationship with a romantic partner during the fifth follow-up period.

Taken together, these results are consistent with those of three small scale, short-term studies of the course of BPD. Modestin and Villiger (1989) studied two groups of former inpatients. They found that borderline patients (22%) were not significantly more likely than comparison subjects with other personality disorders (12%) to report being on disability after a mean of 4.5 years of follow-up. And as noted before, Sandell et al. (1993) found that 34% of borderline patients initially treated in a day hospital reported being on disability 3–10 years after their index admission. Links et al. (1998) found that 30% of former borderline inpatients were receiving disability pensions seven years after their index admission. These authors also found that borderline patients with persistent BPD were more likely to be receiving such a pension than those with remitted BPD (42.3% vs. 20.0%).

The clinical implications of this study are complicated. In terms of vocational functioning, it may be that some borderline patients are so dysfunctional that helping them find a source of income is a reasonable

thing to do for those treating them. It may also be that some borderline patients give up working, reduce their hours, or work "under
the table" in order to receive the associated health insurance benefits
(Medicare and Medicaid) that they need to continue their psychiatric
(and medical) care.

In the former case, vocational counseling may be a useful form of adjunctive treatment and/or the focus of a primary therapy. In the latter case,
a national health insurance system that separates vocational functioning
from access to health care might well be a better model for borderline
patients who can work but are discouraged from doing so under our current system.

In terms of social functioning, about a third of borderline patients who
received SSDI during the course of the study did not have a good relationship with at least one friend during the fifth follow-up period, and about
half did not have a good relationship with a spouse or partner during
this period. Looked at another way, about a third had either no friends
or a conflicted relationship with one or more friends. In a similar vein,
about half either did not have a partner or had a contentious relationship with one. These results suggest that a focus in therapy on the interpersonal functioning of borderline patients receiving disability benefits
would be useful. While this seems obvious, none of the five main forms
of therapy for BPD has been shown to be effective in improving interpersonal functioning—in terms of either forming new relationships or developing less contentious ones (Gunderson & Links, 2008).

In the second of these studies (Zanarini et al., 2010a), 25.9% of borderline patients and 58.3% of Axis II comparison subjects had had good
social and vocational functioning in the two years prior to their index
admission. About 60% of borderline patients and 93% of Axis II comparison subjects who did not have good psychosocial functioning at baseline
achieved this outcome by the time of the 10-year follow-up. In addition,
over 80% of those in both study groups who were high-functioning psychosocially prior to their index admission lost this level of functioning
over the decade of follow-up. And only 40% of borderline patients and

30% of Axis II comparison subjects who lost this level of functioning regained it over the years of follow-up.

To deal with our overly optimistic findings in this area, full-time work or school was now part of the definition of good psychosocial functioning. It was found that almost all cases of losing good psychosocial functioning at baseline or failing to achieve it over time did so because they were unable to function well and in a sustained manner at a full-time job or academic program. This pattern was also true for those with BPD who attained good psychosocial functioning over time but then lost this important outcome.

All of the figures presented here for both study groups would be quite different if we had defined good psychosocial functioning as including part-time work or school (rather than full-time vocational engagement) as we had at six-year follow-up (Zanarini, Frankenburg, Hennen, et al., 2005). With only this one change to our definition, 82% of borderline patients and 94% of Axis II comparison subjects (rather than 60% and 93%) who did not have good psychosocial functioning in the two years prior to their index admission achieved this outcome over the years of follow-up. In a similar vein, 68% of borderline patients and 60% of Axis II comparison subjects (rather than 88% and 84%) who did have good psychosocial functioning at baseline lost it over time. Finally, 81% of borderline patients and 71% of Axis II comparison subjects (rather than 40% and 30%) who lost their initially good psychosocial functioning regained it over time.

It is not clear what interferes with the psychosocial functioning of borderline patients, particularly in the vocational realm. It might be symptoms of BPD. It might also be co-occurring Axis I disorders. Or it might be something temperamental in nature. This temperamental aspect, in turn, could be something specific to BPD or something shared by many people who have trouble achieving and maintaining good social and/or vocational functioning. In addition, this dysfunction could be related to the process of aging. A report from the Collaborative Longitudinal Personality Disorders Study (CLPS) found that the psychosocial functioning of borderline patients who were in their mid-thirties and mid-forties at baseline improved over the first three years of prospective follow-up but started to decline in the latter half of the six years they were followed (Shea et al., 2009).

Two other reports from CLPS found that psychosocial functioning was not an area of strength over time for those with BPD. Skodol et al. (2005) found that those with BPD taken together did not improve psychosocially over two years of prospective follow-up. However, those with BPD who had declining levels of borderline psychopathology did evidence some improvement in this area of functioning. Gunderson, Stout, et al. (2011) found that the overall functioning of those with BPD was basically flat at a relatively low level over 10 years of prospective follow-up.

PSYCHOSOCIAL FUNCTIONING OVER 16 YEARS OF PROSPECTIVE FOLLOW-UP

A third study pertaining to psychosocial functioning was conducted after 16 years of prospective follow-up (Zanarini, Frankenburg, Reich, Wedig, et al., 2015). It pertained to rates of marriage and becoming a parent over the course of the study, including before joining the study. It compared borderline patients who had achieved recovery and those who had not. ("Recovery" was defined as concurrent remission from BPD, and exhibiting good social and good full-time vocational functioning.) It was found that recovered borderline patients were significantly more likely than non-recovered borderline patients to have married/lived with an intimate partner (79% vs. 39%) and to have become a parent (49% vs. 31%). In addition, they first married/cohabited (29 vs. 25) and became a parent (30 vs. 23) at a significantly older age. They were also significantly less likely to have been divorced or ended a cohabiting relationship (42% vs.75%). In addition, they were significantly less likely to have given up or lost custody of a child (7% vs. 51%).

Some clinicians believe that the intimate relationships of most border-line patients end in divorce or a chaotic breakup. They also believe that most borderline patients cannot be good parents. Our results suggest that recovered borderline patients who, as noted, are generally older when marrying or moving in with a romantic partner and when first becoming a parent can achieve stability in these areas.

It is also important to note that even the borderline patients who had trouble parenting stably due to their continuing illness, in most cases voluntarily relinquished custody of their children to a relative rather than having a government agency remove their child or children due to neglect or abuse. In most cases, they visited regularly, and in many cases, their young adult children returned to their home to live—suggesting a somewhat transient difficulty with parenting due to the severity of their illness and resultant psychosocial impairment, rather than an inherent lifelong deficit in these areas.

11

Recovery from Borderline Personality Disorder

A s groundbreaking as our findings concerning the high rates of symptomatic remission and low rates of symptomatic recurrence are, the rates of recovery are even more important. This is so because we defined "recovery" as concurrent symptomatic remission and good social and good full-time vocational functioning (Zanarini et al., 2010b). More specifically, we defined "good social functioning" as having at least one emotionally sustaining relationship with a close friend or life partner/spouse. We defined "good full-time vocational engagement" as being able to work or go to school consistently, competently, and on a full-time basis (i.e., 32 hours or more per week).

Recovery is such an important concept because, if present, it indicates that a person initially diagnosed with BPD has achieved most adult goals in terms of psychosocial functioning as well as a significant reduction in their borderline symptoms—a reduction so great that he or she would no longer be seen as psychiatrically ill with BPD. This concept is also important because it suggests that those achieving it are more productive and perhaps more fulfilled than those who do not achieve it.

Table 11.1 presents the cumulative rates of recovery of two, four, six, and eight years for borderline patients and Axis II comparison subjects (Zanarini et al., 2012).

It is clear that the cumulative rates of recoveries of all lengths increase with time. For example, 14% of borderline patients achieve a two-year recovery by the two-year follow-up, but 60% achieve a two-year recovery by the time of the 16-year follow-up.

It is also clear that the longer the recovery, the lower the rates of recovery. For example, while 60% of borderline patients achieved a two-year

TABLE 11.1   CUMULATIVE RATES OF RECOVERY FOR BORDERLINE PATIENTS AND AXIS II COMPARISON SUBJECTS OVER 16 YEARS OF PROSPECTIVE FOLLOW-UP

	2 YR FU	4 YR FU	6 YR FU	8 YR FU	10 YR FU	12 YR FU	14 YR FU	16 YR FU
Recoveries Lasting 2 Years								
BPD	14	27	36	43	47	50	56	60
OPD	51	67	71	77	84	85	85	85
Recoveries Lasting 4 Years								
BPD		12	24	33	40	44	46	54
OPD		47	63	67	70	77	82	82
Recoveries Lasting 6 Years								
BPD			12	23	31	37	41	44
OPD			43	59	63	68	74	80
Recoveries Lasting 8 Years								
BPD				11	21	28	35	40
OPD				42	57	59	64	75

Percent of recoveries is additive over time

recovery, only 40% achieved an eight-year recovery. In addition, it is clear that Axis II comparison subjects more rapidly achieved a recovery despite its length than borderline patients. For example, 51% of Axis II comparison subjects achieved a two-year recovery by the two-year follow-up, while as mentioned before, only 14% of borderline patients attained this outcome. It is also clear that Axis II comparison subjects do not experience the substantial decline that borderline patients do, when looking at the length of recovery. For example, 85% of comparison subjects achieved a two-year recovery over the course of the study, while 75% achieved an eight-year recovery over the 16 years of prospective follow-up. In sum, borderline patients are substantially less likely to recover from BPD than to experience a symptomatic remission. They are also less likely to recover than Axis II comparison subjects, and they recover at a significantly slower pace.

Table 11.2 presents the cumulative rates of loss of recovery after recoveries of two, four, six, and eight years for borderline patients and Axis II comparison subjects. It should be noted that loss of recoveries is assessed by the number of years that have elapsed since the first recovery, and not at particular time periods as recoveries are assessed.

As can be seen, the shorter the recovery, the higher the rate of loss of recovery. This was true for both groups of subjects. For borderline patients, loss of recoveries was 44% after a two-year recovery, 32% after a four-year recovery, 26% after a six-year recovery, and 20% after an eight-year recovery.

In terms of between-group comparisons, rates of loss of recovery after a two-year recovery were 44% for borderline patients and 28% for Axis II comparison subjects. Rates of loss of recovery after an eight-year recovery were 20% and 9%, respectively.

These findings indicate that it is more difficult for borderline patients to achieve recovery than to achieve symptomatic remission, particularly longer recoveries. These findings also indicate that rates of loss of recoveries were higher than rates of symptomatic recurrences. These findings are also true for Axis II comparison subjects, but to a substantially smaller degree.

TABLE 11.2 CUMULATIVE RATES OF LOSS OF RECOVERY
FOR BORDERLINE PATIENTS AND AXIS II COMPARISON SUBJECTS OVER
16 YEARS OF PROSPECTIVE FOLLOW-UP

	2 YRS After 1st Recovery	4 YRS After 1st Recovery	6 YRS After 1st Recovery	8 YRS After 1st Recovery	10 YRS After 1st Recovery	12 YRS After 1st Recovery	14 YRS After 1st Recovery
			Loss of Recoveries Lasting 2 Years				
BPD	18	25	32	34	37	39	44
OPD	9	17	21	23	28	28	28
			Loss of Recoveries Lasting 4 Years				
BPD	8	16	19	23	26	32	
OPD	8	12	15	20	20	20	
			Loss of Recoveries Lasting 6 Years				
BPD	8	12	17	19	26		
OPD	5	7	13	13	13		
			Loss of Recoveries Lasting 8 Years				
BPD	4	9	12	20			
OPD	3	9	9	9			

Percent of loss of recoveries is additive over time

This set of findings has important clinical implications for borderline
patients, their families, and the mental health professionals working with
them. This is so because achieving and maintaining recovery indicates an
ability to take care of oneself and possibly experience a certain satisfaction
with one's life. The reverse is also probably true. The failure to recover both
symptomatically and psychosocially may well be associated with a continuing dependency on one's family of origin and a continuing high level
of inner pain, particularly feelings of shame that they have not achieved
the life they planned for when younger, and worry that they might end
up all alone with no one to help them or care about them. It can also lead
parents and siblings to worry about what will happen to their child or sibling as he or she ages. Will he or she be alone? How much responsibility

will the parent or sibling have to assume? These concerns are particularly relevant to subjects in the study, who were about 27 years old on average during their index admission, but who are now about 52 (at the partially completed 24-year follow-up).

It is difficult to compare our findings to those of four earlier long-term follow-back studies of the course of BPD, as they did not operationalize their overall outcome beyond what the HSRS or the GAS stated (McGlashan, 1986; Paris et al., 1987; Plakun et al., 1985; Stone, 1990). All four of these studies reported an overall mean score in the 60s a mean of 14–16 years after index admission. However as noted before, two of these studies broke down their overall outcomes further. McGlashan (1986) reported that half of the borderline patients (53%) in the Chestnut Lodge study were functioning in the good–recovered range, while the other half (47%) were functioning in the moderate–incapacitated range. In Stone's New York State Psychiatric Institute study (1990), almost half of the surviving borderline patients received a GAS score in the recovered range (41%), 28% received a GAS score in the good range, 18% in the fair range, and 13% in the marginal–incapacitated range. Our 60% recovery figure is about halfway between McGlashan's 53% and Stone's 69%, but consistent with both.

In terms of prospective long-term studies of the overall outcome of BPD, the CLPS study (Gunderson, Stout, et al., 2011) used a GAF score of 71 or higher, while our operationalized criteria were tied to a GAF score of 61 or higher. We used this score to be consistent with the older follow-back studies. A GAF score in this range is described as having "some mild symptoms or some difficulty in social, occupational, or school functioning but generally functioning pretty well, has some meaningful interpersonal relationships." However, a GAF score in the 71–80 range is described as: "If symptoms are present, they are transient and expectable reactions to psychosocial stressors; no more than slight impairment in social, occupational, or school functioning." Using this stringent definition, somewhat less than 25% of the borderline patients in the CLPS study achieved this outcome after 10 years of prospective follow-up. And the mean GAF score of these borderline patients only improved over the decade of the study from 53 to 57—a score in the "fair" range of symptom severity and functioning.

Plainly, there is a difference between patients with BPD who only remit, and those who also recover. Following are two vignettes detailing these differences in background and course.

MS. C: REMISSION WITHOUT RECOVERY

Upon study entry, Ms. C was a 28-year-old single white female from a seemingly stable working class family. She had functioned well throughout college, but become very symptomatic after graduation. She repeatedly engaged in self-harm and made suicide attempts. While close to her parents, she was very demanding of them. She was also very anxious, lonely, and empty. While in college, she had been somewhat promiscuous and had abused alcohol on weekends. She was preoccupied with abandonment concerns and had a pattern of treatment regressions.

Prior to her index admission, she had had a very intense psychotherapy with a therapist with whom she quickly developed a dependent relationship. She stayed in this therapy for six years and began to function more poorly in the world of work, although she was working regularly at a part-time job and living on her own.

During her index admission, she first reported a childhood history of sexual abuse by male relatives when she was in late latency. She stated that she had always remembered this abuse but had not mentioned it for fear it would hurt her family. Her hospital team suggested that she terminate with her current therapist and start to see a trauma expert. This therapist focused almost exclusively on Ms. C's trauma history, and the more she focused on it, the worse Ms. C felt and functioned. She was repeatedly hospitalized for self-harm, suicide threats and attempts, and ever deepening depressive episodes. This pattern continued for about four years. Ms. C's initial competence was "forgotten," and she was seen as a chronic patient who had never done well and who would never do well. In fact, her symptoms were so severe and her psychosocial functioning was so tenuous that she started to support herself on Social Security disability payments. She no longer had any friends, never dated, and was no longer working due to crippling anxiety at work. In addition, she moved into supportive housing.

After a consultation, Ms. C who was highly intelligent, started to be seen in a supportive psychotherapy that did not deal with her abuse history but focused on her difficulty functioning on a day-to-day basis. Despite this therapist's best efforts, Ms. C became housebound, did not make friends, did not try to date, and completely gave up on getting a job or doing almost anything outside her apartment. However, with this supportive approach, many of Ms. C's symptoms abated, and she has not been hospitalized since 10-year follow-up.

Ms. C is currently only symptomatic in the areas of experiential avoidance and undue dependency. She is chronically anxious, particularly outside her apartment, and avoids all situations that make her anxious. Despite apparent competence, she is now basically housebound except for psychiatric and medical appointments. However, she has adapted to her situation by developing a number of hobbies that she can pursue on her own. She is a voracious reader, enjoys painting, and has adopted a pet that she is very fond of and seems to meet some of her needs for closeness.

She has continued to see her therapist once a week and is still seeing her original psychiatrist, who has prescribed very aggressive polypharmacy for her over the years. She is not sure if this regimen is helpful but wants to continue her relationship with this physician as she finds it supportive.

Over the years, she has gained 70 pounds and is now morbidly obese. Very few of those who know her now remember that she was normal weight at study entrance. She suffers from fibromyalgia, gastrointestinal reflux disease (GERD), high blood pressure, high cholesterol, and type 2 diabetes. She is receiving treatment for each of these disorders and is compliant with treatment recommendations, except for losing weight and becoming more physically active. She is also taking an opioid pain medication for her fibromyalgia and reports that she has not increased the dose on her own.

Ms. C remitted at 12-year follow-up and has not had a recurrence. However, she has never recovered, as she has been without friends or a significant other. In addition, she has not been able to work consistently, competently, and on a full-time basis.

Why did it take her so long to remit? Why has she never recovered? In terms of remission, one might point to her trauma history and/or the intensive forms of treatment she received before working with her current supportive therapist. And one or both of these factors might be implicated in this outcome. In terms of recovery, the intensity of her first therapy after her index admission may have taken much of her emotional energy that could have gone to making friends, dating, and working. However, her extreme experiential avoidance and dependency may have strongly interfered with achieving these milestones of adulthood. In addition, her multiple hospitalizations lent an air of instability to her life, as it was never clear if she was going to be living at home or in the hospital for a time.

MS. D: BOTH REMISSION AND RECOVERY

Ms. D was an 18-year-old single white female. She came from an intact middle class family. Both her parents were college graduates who were gainfully employed. She had one younger sibling. She reported feeling emotionally ill at the age of 16, first entered treatment at the age of 18, and had her first psychiatric hospitalization at this age as well.

She also reported that she did not have a family history of psychiatric disorder, her parents were competent in most areas, and that she had been competent both in latency and adolescence. She denied any childhood abuse or neglect.

She was a freshman at a local college and complained of mounting feelings of homesickness and depression. She had started to hear a voice telling her to hurt herself. Despite knowing that it was probably her own thoughts, she repeatedly cut and burned herself. She also had trouble making friends at college and relied on her parents and one friend from high school for social support. She managed to get good grades her first semester but started to falter academically her second semester. Her parents encouraged her to see someone at the college mental health center. Upon meeting with Ms. D, the social worker doing the intake felt that she was acutely suicidal and recommended that she be hospitalized until these symptoms lessened in intensity.

After a hospitalization of several weeks, her depression lessened somewhat in response to having more support and structure as well as starting to take an antidepressant. She and her parents decided she should take a leave from college and move home. Once there, she became increasingly anxious as well as angry at and demanding of her parents' time and attention. She blamed them for not preparing her to be independent and often repeated a litany of complaints that she insisted they hear. Given the seriousness and changing nature of her symptoms, Ms. D entered outpatient psychotherapy for the first time and continued seeing her hospital psychiatrist for medication.

In therapy, she talked about strong feelings of self-hatred, depersonalization, and emptiness. She was also ashamed about how dependent she was on her family and how angry she was for their failure to help her separate from them, blaming them for her failure at college. Gradually, her depression lessened, she stopped having command hallucinations, and she stopped hurting herself physically. However, she entered her first serious relationship with a young man whom she knew from high school, but the relationship soon turned stormy as she felt abandoned when he went to work or wanted to spend time with his friends.

Eventually, she got a part-time job at the local public library and found that she liked this type of work, as the environment was academic but supportive. She continued in outpatient therapy and worked on her feelings of dysphoria and worthlessness as well as her abandonment concerns and anger at and blaming of her parents, who now attended psychotherapy with her once a month.

After seven months of outpatient treatment, she returned to college but continued to live at home and see the same treatment team. She broke off the relationship with her boyfriend as she thought it stirred up too many feelings that she could not handle. Her demands on her parents lessened as she made two close friends at college. She switched her major from history to library science and did well in her course work. She graduated with honors and enrolled in a master's program in library science. She was still living at home but no longer was symptomatic in any areas except for dependency, which she recognized was a problem and about which she felt ashamed. In her second year, she met an engineering student and started dating him. Like her, he was reserved and dutiful. After several months, they moved in together. Ms. D now realized how much support her parents had given her over the years and began to express her gratitude to them in many ways. She realized that she had been blaming them for a dependency that was hers since early childhood.

After she graduated, she got a job as a librarian in the suburb in which she grew up and in which her parents still lived. Her boyfriend was now settled in a job as a civil engineer that he liked and where he felt that his work was respected. They got married a year later and bought a home near her parents. Three years later, they had their only child, a son. They both continued to work full-time, and her mother took care of her son during the work week.

She continued to see her two friends from college on a monthly basis and to exercise daily by jogging with her husband. Her physical health was excellent and her husband and son were both thriving at work and school, respectively. After 10 years with her therapist, she was able to terminate with the proviso that she could return at any time if she thought it necessary. She expressed gratitude to her therapist for helping her grow up. However, she continued to see her psychiatrist for medication checks once a month, saying "I do not know if this antidepressant is working but I am afraid to go off it and get so sick again."

Ms. D achieved remission at four-year follow-up and never had a symptomatic recurrence. She achieved recovery at the same time period as she had several emotionally supportive relationships outside her family of origin (e.g., two close friends she saw on a daily basis) and was able to go the school consistently, competently, and on a full-time basis. She never lost this recovery, and in fact it deepened with her marriage, motherhood, and her satisfying full-time work as one of several town librarians.

Why was she able to achieve remission and recovery relatively rapidly and stably? While it is impossible to know, her family was supportive of her and did not have noted psychopathology. Ms. D was achievement-oriented and determined to succeed. While a reserved person, she was not so hampered socially that she was prevented from making friends and marrying someone who respected her and was supportive of her. Additionally, she was able to remain with the same therapist for a decade in once-a-week supportive therapy, and the therapy was never so intense that a regression ensued.

12

Predictors of Time-to-Remission and Recovery

For both time-to-remission and recovery outcomes, 10 families of predictors were studied, encompassing 40 to 41 baseline predictors. These families of predictors were: demographic characteristics, treatment history, pathological childhood experiences, protective childhood experiences, family history of psychiatric disorder, lifetime Axis I disorders, co-occurring Axis II disorders, aspects of normal temperament, aspects of adult competence (in the two years prior to index admission), and adverse adult experiences. We first studied predictors of time-to-remission at 10-year follow-up (Zanarini, Frankenburg, Hennen, Reich, & Silk, 2006). We then studied predictors of time-to-recovery at 16-year follow-up (Zanarini, Frankenburg, Reich, et al., 2014). In each of these specific studies, we began by testing the significance of each predictor separately. We then put all of the significant predictors of that outcome together in a multivariable model.

PREDICTION OF TIME-TO-REMISSION

Table 12.1 lists all of the baseline variables used to predict time-to-remission by 10-year follow-up, which was achieved by 88% of those with BPD (and not the 99% who achieved this goal by the time of the 16-year follow-up) (Zanarini et al., 2010b). The first column contains the predictors that were significant predictors, and the second column contains the predictors were non-significant.

As can be seen, 16 variables were significant predictors in themselves, while 24 predictors were non-significant taken by themselves. The significant predictors encompassed nine families of baseline predictors (all but "adult adversity"). More specifically, these families encompassed the following variables: demographic characteristics (25 or younger), treatment history (no prior hospitalizations), pathological childhood experiences (absence of sexual abuse, severity of other forms of abuse, severity of neglect, severity of witnessed violence), protective childhood experiences (degree of childhood competence), family history of psychiatric disorder (no mood disorder in family, no substance use disorder in family), lifetime Axis I disorders (absence of PTSD), co-occurring Axis II disorders (absence of anxious cluster disorder), aspects of normal temperament (neuroticism, extraversion, agreeableness, and conscientiousness), and aspects of adult competence (good premorbid vocational/academic record).

When viewed more synthetically, two predictors suggested a lack of chronicity (age 25 or younger and no prior hospitalizations), four were forms of childhood adversity (absence of sexual abuse, severity of other forms of abuse, severity of neglect, and severity of witnessed violence), two represent competence (degree of childhood competence and good adult vocational/academic record), two are disorders "running" in families (no mood or substance use disorder in family), co-occurring disorders (absence of PTSD and absence of anxious cluster personality disorder), and four factors of normal temperament (neuroticism, extraversion, agreeableness, and conscientiousness).

Box 12.1 details the significant multivariable baseline predictors of time-to-remission at 10 years of follow-up.

TABLE 12.1 BASELINE PREDICTORS OF TIME-TO-REMISSION

Significant Predictors	Non-Significant Predictors
25 Years Old or Younger at Index Admission (median age = 26)	Female
No Prior Hospitalization	White
Absence of Sexual Abuse	Age of Onset of Symptoms
Severity of Other Forms of Abuse	Age of First Treatment
Severity of Neglect	Early Childhood Separations
Severity of Witnessed Violence	No Parental Divorce
Degree of Childhood Competence	Number of Positive Relationships in Childhood
No Mood Disorder in Family	Degree of Parental Competence
No Substance Use Disorder in Family	Higher IQ
Lifetime Absence of PTSD	No Anxiety Disorder in Family
Absence of Anxious Cluster Disorder	No Eating Disorder in Family
Lower Neuroticism	No Dramatic Cluster Disorder in Family
Higher Extraversion	Lifetime Absence of Mood Disorder
Higher Agreeableness	Lifetime Absence of Substance Use Disorder
Higher Conscientiousness	Lifetime Absence of Another Anxiety Disorder
Good Vocational Record	Lifetime Absence of Eating Disorder
	Absence of Odd Cluster Disorder
	Absence of Non-BPD Dramatic Cluster Disorder
	Higher Openness
	Good Relationship with Partner
	Good Relationship with Parent(s)
	Number of Friends
	No Adult Rape History
	No Physically Violent Partner

Box 12.1   **MULTIVARIATE BASELINE PREDICTORS OF**
TIME-TO-REMISSION

Baseline DIB-R Score

Age 25 or Younger

Good Premorbid Vocational Record

No History of Childhood Sexual Abuse

No Family History of Substance Abuse

Absence of Co-occurring Anxious Cluster Axis II Disorder

Lower Neuroticism Score

Higher Agreeableness Score

As can be seen here, seven of the 16 significant predictors remain in this model controlling for severity of borderline psychopathology at baseline (as represented by the total DIB-R score). These variables were: younger age, absence of childhood sexual abuse, no family history of substance use disorder, good vocational/academic record, absence of an anxious cluster personality disorder, lower neuroticism, and higher agreeableness. In terms of specific variables, the association of younger age with earlier time-to-remission runs counter to the clinical lore of BPD (and other psychiatric disorders), where getting older is believed to lead to a lessening of symptomatic impairment. However, it makes clinical sense that younger people do better symptomatically, as they may not yet be hampered by life mistakes and are probably less likely to be chronic patients.

Not having a personal history of being sexually abused as a child or a family history of substance abuse also make clinical sense as predictors of a good symptomatic outcome, as they suggest a childhood less marred by trauma and turmoil. In addition, a stable work or school history was a strong multivariate predictor of time-to-remission. This suggests that adult competence in the psychosocial realm is important for symptomatic improvement. This may be because these patients struggle harder to get better, or at least may be less attached to the patient role. It may also be that they are more innately competent than borderline patients who do more poorly.

The triad of temperamental predictors suggests that a higher level of agreeableness is helpful in getting better symptomatically, while a higher level of neuroticism and avoidant, dependent, obsessive-compulsive, and self-defeating personality traits makes it harder to get well. This, too, makes clinical sense. Neuroticism, while an aspect of normal personality, is also a compilation of symptomatic states, such as anger, anxiety, and depression. Clearly, those borderline patients burdened with a higher degree of these states or traits would have a harder time making symptomatic progress. In a similar manner, borderline patients burdened by being shy, dependent, unduly perfectionistic, and masochistic might have a harder time making the effort to get well. However, borderline patients who are endowed with a more affiliative or agreeable personality (e.g., not being particularly argumentative or manipulative) may have an easier time getting other people to support and assist them emotionally. This, in turn, could be crucial to the process of getting better symptomatically, as it could ameliorate the abandonment concerns that tend to intensify for borderline patients as progress is being made.

These results suggest that prediction of symptomatic outcome for BPD is multifactorial. It encompasses predictors that are routinely assessed in clinical practice because of their clinical importance, such as childhood history of sexual abuse and family history of substance use disorders. It also encompasses predictors that are commonly discussed in treatment but may not receive the attention that they deserve, such as stage of adult development and adult competence. Finally, prediction of time-to-remission seems to encompass aspects of temperament, such as low levels of shyness and undue dependency, which are probably noticed but rarely discussed in clinical practice.

PREDICTION OF TIME-TO-RECOVERY

The only information on predictors of the overall outcome of BPD prior to MSAD comes from the four large-scale, long-term, follow-back studies that were conducted in the 1980s (McGlashan, 1986; Paris et al., 1987; Plakun et al., 1985; Stone, 1990).

Each of these studies tried to determine the best predictors of general outcome a mean of 14–16 years after index admission. Five factors were found to be associated with a good long-term outcome: high IQ (McGlashan, 1985; Stone, 1990), being unusually talented or physically attractive (if female) (Stone, 1990), the absence of parental divorce and narcissistic entitlement (Plakun, 1991), and the presence of physically self-destructive acts during the index admission (McGlashan, 1985). Nine factors were found to be associated with a poor long-term outcome: affective instability (McGlashan, 1985), chronic dysphoria (Paris et al., 1987), younger age at first treatment (Paris et al., 1987), length of prior hospitalization (McGlashan, 1985), antisocial behavior (Stone, 1990), substance abuse (Stone, 1990), parental brutality (Stone, 1990), a family history of psychiatric illness (Paris et al., 1987), and a problematic relationship with one's mother (but not one's father) (Paris, Nowlis, & Brown, 1988).

Table 12.2 lists all of the baseline variables used to predict time-to-recovery after 16 years of prospective follow-up, an outcome that was achieved, as noted elsewhere, by 60% of those with BPD. These variables are the same as the potential predictors of time-to-remission, with the addition of no ADHD.

The results are the same, too—with the following exceptions: higher IQ, absence of odd cluster personality disorder, number of friends (in past two years), and no ADHD are now significant bivariate predictors of time-to-recovery. However, three factors are now non-significant bivariate predictors of this outcome: absence of sexual abuse in childhood, no mood disorder in family, and trait conscientiousness. All told, 17 variables were significant predictors and 24 were non-significant predictors of time-to-recovery.

All families of predictors were represented in the significant bivariate predictors of time-to-recovery, except for experiences of adult adversity (as was true for significant bivariate predictors of time-to-remission). Thus, factors pertaining to demographics, treatment history, adverse childhood experiences, protective childhood experiences, family history of

TABLE 12.2   BASELINE PREDICTORS OF TIME-TO-RECOVERY

Significant Predictors	Non-Significant Predictors
25 Years Old or Younger at Index Admission (median age = 26)	Female
No Prior Hospitalization	White
Severity of Other Forms of Abuse	Age of Onset of Symptoms
Severity of Neglect	Age of First Treatment
Severity of Witnessed Violence	Absence of Sexual Abuse
Degree of Childhood Competence	Early Childhood Separations
Higher IQ	No Parental Divorce
No ADHD	Number of Positive Relationships in Childhood
No Substance Use Disorder in Family	Degree of Parental Competence
Lifetime Absence of PTSD	No Mood Disorder in Family
Absence of Odd Cluster Disorder	No Anxiety Disorder in Family
Absence of Anxious Cluster Disorder	No Eating Disorder in Family
Lower Neuroticism	No Dramatic Cluster Disorder in Family
Higher Extraversion	Lifetime Absence of Mood Disorder
Higher Agreeableness	Lifetime Absence of Substance Use Disorder
Good Vocational Record	Lifetime Absence of Another Anxiety Disorder
Number of Friends	Lifetime Absence of Eating Disorder
	Absence of Non-BPD Dramatic Cluster Disorder
	Higher Openness
	Higher Conscientiousness
	Good Relationship with Partner
	Good Relationship with Parent(s)
	No Adult Rape History
	No Physically Violent Partner

psychiatric disorder, co-occurring Axis I disorders, Axis II co-occurrence, facets of normal personality, and psychosocial functioning in the two years prior to index admission were all found to have a significant relationship to time-to-recovery. More specifically, 17 of the predictor variables that were studied were found to significantly predict earlier time-to-recovery after controlling for baseline severity (represented by GAF score). One of these predictors is demographic (younger age), while another pertains to treatment history (no prior psychiatric hospitalizations). Three are from the adverse childhood experiences family of predictors (less severe childhood abuse of a verbal/emotional/physical nature, less severe childhood neglect [which is mostly emotional], less severe violence witnessed as a child), three pertain to childhood protective factors (higher degree of childhood competence, higher IQ, and the absence of ADHD), and one pertains to family history of psychiatric disorder (no family history of substance use disorder). Three are co-occurring disorders (absence of PTSD, absence of odd cluster personality disorders, and absence of anxious cluster personality disorders), and three are aspects of normal personality (lower neuroticism and higher extraversion and higher agreeableness). Finally, two are elements of recent psychosocial functioning (a good full-time vocational record and number of friends).

The variables that were not found to be significant in these bivariate analyses are also interesting because of their presumed clinical importance (e.g., gender, early childhood separations, childhood sexual abuse) and the fact that some of them (e.g., younger age at first treatment, substance abuse, absence of parental divorce) have been found to be significant predictors of outcome in follow-back studies of the long-term course of BPD (Paris et al., 1987; Stone, 1990; Plakun, 1991).

The lack of a significant bivariate relationship between childhood sexual abuse and time-to-recovery is probably the most important of these factors. Many clinicians believe that a history of childhood sexual abuse leads to the development of key symptoms of BPD (Herman & van der Kolk, 1987). Some clinicians also believe that this type of abuse in childhood makes it very difficult, if not impossible, for someone to function effectively as an adult. The results of this study suggest that this may not be true for all borderline patients with such a history. In fact, the severity of other forms of childhood abuse, the severity of neglect, and the severity of witnessed violence all were significant bivariate predictors of time-to-recovery—suggesting that they play a more pronounced role in the overall symptomatic and functional outcome of those with BPD than a childhood history of sexual abuse. Or, looked at in another way, childhood sexual abuse may well play a role in the development of BPD, but it does not seem to directly play a role in recovery from BPD—which, as noted here, seems more related to innate endowment or temperamental factors.

Box 12.2 details the significant multivariable baseline predictors of time-to-recovery by 16 years of follow-up.

In terms of significant multivariate predictors, six of the bivariate predictors remained significant after controlling for overall baseline severity: no prior psychiatric hospitalizations, higher IQ, good vocational record, absence of an anxious cluster personality disorder, higher extraversion, and higher agreeableness. In terms of specific variables, one is associated with a lack of chronicity: no prior psychiatric hospitalizations. It is not surprising that borderline patients who have never been hospitalized before would have a better prognosis than borderline patients with a history of multiple hospitalizations. However, this finding may also represent a cohort effect, as the length of hospitalizations shortened dramatically as the study was beginning, and their purpose changed from emotional

---

Box 12.2 MULTIVARIATE BASELINE PREDICTORS OF TIME-TO-RECOVERY

Baseline GAF Score
No Prior Psychiatric Hospitalizations
Good Vocational Record
Higher IQ
Absence of Co-occurring Anxious Cluster Axis II Disorder
Higher Extraversion Score
Higher Agreeableness Score

growth to symptom stabilization—both of which probably lessened the chances of a serious regression.

Two other variables are associated with competence: a higher IQ and a stable work or school history in the two years prior to index admission. Being more intelligent may make it easier to put the past in perspective, or at least enhance one's chances of learning new ways of coping with old grievances and seemingly ingrained maladaptive patterns. Having a steady vocational record in the two years prior to index admission suggests a greater likelihood of having the ability to work or go to school competently, consistently, and on a full-time basis over the years of follow-up, which is part of our definition of recovery, than someone who never had such a record or who had such a record of vocational achievement but relinquished it more than two years ago.

The final three variables associated with an earlier time-to-recovery are aspects of temperament: being without the avoidance and dependency of anxious cluster personality disorders, as well as exhibiting higher levels of extraversion and agreeableness. In the five-factor model, "extraversion" includes positive emotions as well as being outgoing, while "agreeableness" includes being cooperative as well as compassionate (Costa & McCrae, 1992).

All three of these temperamental predictors suggest an easier path to fulfilling our definition of good social functioning—having a stable relationship with a close friend or spouse/life partner—than being avoidant, introverted, and/or prone to aggravation at the slightest disappointment or disagreement. All three may also make it easier to achieve a good vocational record—another part of our definition of recovery. Many borderline patients avoid getting a job or going to school, particularly on a full-time basis, because they fear that it will make them too anxious or overwhelmed. And being more outgoing makes it easier to deal with the interpersonal aspects of work or school. In addition, being more understanding of others may well lead to less conflict at work or school and opens the door to the possibility that this arena of functioning could lead to new sustaining relationships as well as a sense of accomplishment. In any event, full-time work or school provides structure to one's life and some degree, however limited, of social interaction.

The "families" of predictors that did not contribute to our multivariate model of factors associated with recovery are also telling: demography, childhood adversity, family history of psychiatric disorder, Axis I psychopathology, and adult adversity or experiences of violence as an adult. As noted before, both the absence of childhood sexual abuse and the absence of a family history of substance use disorder were found to be significant multivariate predictors of time-to-remission from BPD after 10 years of prospective follow-up (Zanarini, Frankenburg, Hennen, et al., 2006). It may be that these factors are less relevant to recovery than to remission. It may also be that their effect is attenuated after six additional years of follow-up.

The overall take-home message of this study is that time-to-recovery is more related to enduring attributes that borderline patients may have than to things that were done to them or things that were not done for them; nor to the Axis I pathology they suffered from, nor disorders that "ran" in their families through genetics, social learning, or some combination of the two.

The results of this study suggest that intelligence and industriousness, coupled with a more outgoing and empathic and less avoidant nature, may form the foundation upon which recovery rests. Yet, as we have noted before, none of the five comprehensive empirically based treatments for BPD are aimed at these factors (Zanarini et al., 2007). In terms of remediation, we have suggested developing treatments focused on helping borderline patients learn to cope with temperamental symptoms or aspects of their personalities that are less than helpful (Zanarini et al., 2007). We have also suggested a rehabilitation model for borderline patients who cannot get a job or stay in school (Zanarini et al., 2012). And this is the crux of the matter, as we have previously found that the inability to work or go to school productively and on a full-time basis is the strongest reason for failure to achieve recovery, or its loss for those with BPD (Zanarini et al., 2010b).

In many ways, these results are sobering as they stress inborn abilities or aspects of temperament rather than adverse events that may have occurred or co-occurring illnesses that may have been experienced personally or in one's family. It is of course possible that these events and psychiatric disorders, such as childhood sexual abuse or PTSD, may have shaped the expression of one's abilities or negatively impacted one's temperament prior to index admission. In any case, patients, family members, and clinicians will have to work together to help the person with BPD to "get around" these factors if treatments are not available that focus on resilience in work or school or provide assistance in altering the expression of one's temperament just enough that it does not present a problem going forward. No one expects shy people to suddenly become outgoing, but perhaps they can work on lessening the severity of the experiential avoidance that may be holding them back vocationally and socially. In a like manner, no one expects everyone with BPD to rapidly become very cooperative and compassionate, but perhaps they may be amenable to handling things just differently enough that they get along with others more smoothly.

In addition, four recent studies have found that BPD and its four constituent sectors of psychopathology or the nine symptoms of BPD are highly heritable (Gunderson, Zanarini, et al., 2011; Kendler et al., 2011; Reichborn-Kjennerud et al., 2013; Torgersen et al., 2012). This heritability may have partially underpinned some of the predictors of recovery that were found to be significant in multivariate analyses. For example, the heritability of interpersonal factors related to BPD may be related inversely to the absence of avoidant features and the higher levels of extraversion and agreeableness that were found to be strongly associated with time-to-recovery from BPD.

13

Co-occurring Disorders over Time

AXIS I DISORDERS OVER SIX YEARS OF PROSPECTIVE FOLLOW-UP

Co-occurring Axis I and II disorders were assessed over six years of prospective follow-up. At baseline, the lifetime rates of all types of Axis I disorders were high: mood disorders, mostly unipolar (97%); substance use disorders (62%); anxiety disorders, including PTSD (89%); and eating disorders (54%) (Zanarini, Frankenburg, Hennen, Reich, & Silk, 2004). Borderline patients experienced declining rates of many Axis I disorders over time. However, the rates of these disorders remained quite high, particularly the rates of mood (75%) and anxiety disorders (60%). We also compared the rates of the 70% of border-line patients who had experienced a two-year symptomatic remission (or one follow-up period) versus the 30% who had not. It was found that remitted borderline patients experienced substantial decline in all concurrent disorders assessed, while those who had not remitted reported stable rates of co-occurring disorders. More specifically, the following rates were found at six-year follow-up: mood disorders (70% vs. 92%), substance use disorders (12% vs. 41%), PTSD (23% vs. 72%), other anxiety disorders (50% vs. 94%), and eating disorders (26% vs. 58%). However, when the absence of these comorbid disorders was used to predict time-to-remission, substance use disorders were a substantially stronger predictor of remission than PTSD, mood disorders, other anxiety disorders, and eating disorders, respectively. Those without a history of a substance use disorder over time were four times more likely to remit (and to remit more rapidly) than those with such a history.

This finding runs counter to clinical lore, which suggests that BPD is most affected by the course of mood disorders or PTSD. However, this finding makes clinical sense, as abusing alcohol and/or drugs could easily lead to greater impairment in all four core sectors of borderline psychopathology: decreased mood, heightened distrust, increased impulsivity, and even more turbulent relationships.

In general, the relationship between remission from BPD and the co-occurrence of one or more Axis I disorders is unclear. It might be that borderline patients who are likely to remit have less Axis I psychopathology initially. However, the baseline rates of all but PTSD (53% vs. 71%) were almost identical for borderline patients who attained a remission from BPD and those who did not. It might be that borderline patients who remit are more responsive to treatment than those who do not. It may also be that there is something fundamentally different about the temperament and/or neurobiology of the two groups of patients.

While high rates of co-occurring disorders are found in many psychiatric disorders, particularly in patients with very high initial acuity, this pattern can be seen as a useful marker for BPD (Zanarini et al., 1998b). Almost 20 years ago, we developed the concept of "complex comorbidity." The operational definition of complex comorbidity is that a patient has met the *DSM* criteria for a broadly defined disorder of affect (a mood disorder *and* an anxiety disorder) and meets *DSM* criteria for a disorder of impulsivity (a substance use disorder or an eating disorder, or both). Overall, a significantly higher percentage of borderline patients than comparison subjects met *DSM* criteria for a combination of disorders of affect and impulsivity (73% versus 27%). The same pattern of comorbidity was found to be discriminating for female borderline and female comparison subjects (76% vs. 34%) as well as for male borderline and male comparison subjects (65% vs. 18%).

AXIS II DISORDERS OVER SIX YEARS
OF PROSPECTIVE FOLLOW-UP

After six years of prospective follow-up, we compared rates of Axis II disorders between remitted and non-remitted borderline patients (Zanarini, Frankenburg, Vujanovic, et al., 2004). Anxious cluster disorders were more common among those in both groups than odd cluster disorders and non-BPD dramatic cluster disorders. Both remitted and non-remitted borderline patients experienced declining rates of most types of Axis II disorders over time. However, the rates of avoidant, dependent, and self-defeating personality disorders and anxious cluster disorders in general remained high among non-remitted borderline patients (85% at baseline and 77% at six-year follow-up). Additionally, the absence of these three disorders was found to be significantly correlated with a borderline patient's likelihood-of-remission and time-to-remission: self-defeating personality disorder by a factor of 4, dependent personality disorder by a factor of 3.5, and avoidant personality disorder by a factor of almost 2. These findings make clinical sense, as being shy and anxious, dependent on others, and engaging in masochistic behaviors all interfere with attaining a prolonged remission of BPD symptoms.

AXIS I DISORDERS OVER 10 YEARS
OF PROSPECTIVE FOLLOW-UP

In a series of studies, we examined prevalence rates of substance use disorders (Zanarini, Frankenburg, et al., 2011), PTSD (Zanarini, Hörz, et al., 2011), other anxiety disorders (Silverman, Frankenburg, Reich, Fitzmaurice, & Zanarini, 2012), and eating disorders (Zanarini, Reichman, Frankenburg, Reich, & Fitzmaurice, 2010) over 10 years of prospective follow-up. We also studied time-to-remission and time-to-recurrence (for those who had the disorder at baseline) as well as time-to-new-onsets (for those who did not have the disorder at baseline).

DISORDERS OF IMPULSE OVER A DECADE
OF PROSPECTIVE FOLLOW-UP

Here we report the results for substance use disorders (SUDs) and eating disorders (EDs), as both involve a degree of volition and impulsivity.

Substance Use Disorders

The prevalence of SUDs among borderline patients and Axis II comparison subjects declined significantly over time, while remaining significantly more common among those with BPD. More specifically, the rate of alcohol abuse/dependence declined from 50% to 9%, while the rate of drug abuse/dependence declined from 47% to 7%. In terms of time-to-event results, over 90% of borderline patients meeting criteria for a SUD at baseline experienced a remission by 10-year follow-up (92% alcohol and 95% drugs). Recurrences (35% drugs and 40% alcohol) and new onsets of SUDs were less common (21% drugs and 23% alcohol). Taken together, these results present a more positive clinical picture for SUDS than commonly recognized. Remissions seem relatively stable, and new onsets are not that common. However, over the subsequent years of the study, this picture may shift as our subjects enter middle age and with it, greater responsibilities, stress, and lack of social supports.

Eating Disorders

The prevalence of anorexia, bulimia, and eating disorder not otherwise specified (EDNOS) declined significantly over time for those in both study groups but the prevalence of EDNOS remained significantly higher among borderline patients than among participants with other Axis II disorders. More specifically, the following baseline and 10-year prevalence rates were found for borderline patients: anorexia (22% and 2%), bulimia (21% and 2), and EDNOS (28% to 17%).

In terms of time-to-event data, over 90% of borderline patients meeting criteria for anorexia, bulimia, or EDNOS at baseline experienced a stable remission by the time of the 10-year follow-up. Both recurrences (52%) and new onsets (43%) of EDNOS were more common among borderline patients than recurrences and new onsets of anorexia (28% and 4%) and bulimia (29% and 11%). In addition, diagnostic migration was most common among borderline patients meeting criteria for anorexia at baseline (88%), followed by those meeting criteria for bulimia (71%) and EDNOS (20%), respectively. The results of this study suggest that the prognosis for both anorexia and bulimia in borderline patients is complicated, with remissions being stable but migrations to other eating disorders being common. The results also suggest that EDNOS may be the most prevalent and enduring of the eating disorders in these patients.

An earlier study of the MSAD sample found that binge eating disorder (BED) was the most common form of EDNOS reported at baseline (Marino & Zanarini, 2001). And it is our impression that BED is the most common form of EDNOS over time.

PTSD OVER 10 YEARS OF FOLLOW-UP

The prevalence of PTSD, which was significantly more common among borderline patients at baseline, declined significantly over time for patients with BPD (from 58% to 21%) and for Axis II comparison subjects (from 25% to 3%). Over 85% of borderline patients meeting criteria for PTSD at baseline experienced a remission by the time of the 10-year follow-up. Recurrences (40%) and new onsets (27%) were less common.

In terms of predictors of time-to-remission of PTSD among patients with BPD, it was found in this study that the presence of childhood sexual abuse and the severity of that abuse were both significant predictors. More specifically, patients with a childhood history of sexual abuse were only half as likely to have a remission from PTSD when compared to those without such a history. For each five-point increase of the severity of childhood sexual abuse (on a scale of 0–19), the likelihood of remission of PTSD declined by about 21%.

In terms of sexual adversity occurring during the years of follow-up, it was found that those borderline patients who reported being sexually assaulted during the 10 years of prospective follow-up were almost 11 times more likely to experience a recurrence of PTSD than those who were not sexually assaulted during this decade. Taken together, the results of this study suggest that PTSD is not a chronic disorder for the majority of borderline patients. They also suggest a strong relationship between sexual adversity in both childhood and adulthood and the course of PTSD among patients with BPD.

OTHER ANXIETY DISORDERS OVER A DECADE OF FOLLOW-UP

A significantly higher percentage of borderline patients than Axis II comparison subjects reported experiencing any anxiety disorder other than PTSD, panic disorder, agoraphobia, social phobia, obsessive-compulsive disorder (OCD), and generalized anxiety disorder (GAD) (but not simple phobia). For both borderline patients and Axis II comparison subjects, the rates of anxiety disorders, with the exception of OCD and GAD, declined significantly over time. As an example, about 80% of borderline patients (and about 49% of Axis II comparison subjects) had a history of any anxiety disorder other than PTSD at the time of their index admission. Borderline patients were nearly two times more likely to report experiencing any anxiety disorder other than PTSD as Axis II comparison subjects. And the chance of experiencing any anxiety disorder other than PTSD over the course of the study for those in both groups decreased by 53%.

All six disorders had high rates of remission by the tenth year of follow-up. The rates of remission for borderline patients who met criteria for these anxiety disorders at baseline were as follows: 77% for OCD, 82% for panic disorder, 92% for simple phobia, 97% for social phobia, and 100% for GAD and agoraphobia.

By the time of the 10-year follow-up, 65% of the borderline patients who had remitted from panic disorder and 40% who had remitted from social phobia reported meeting criteria for a recurrence. However, less than 40% of borderline patients who reported a remission of agoraphobia, simple phobia, OCD, or GAD later reported a recurrence of these disorders.

The rates of new onsets of the studied anxiety disorders among borderline patients who had not reported meeting criteria for them at baseline are as follows: 15% for agoraphobia, 17% for OCD, 23% for GAD, 24% for social phobia, 36% for simple phobia, and over 45% for panic disorder. While panic disorder had a high cumulative rate of remission among borderline patients, recurrences and new onsets were common. These results suggest that panic disorder may be the most problematic anxiety disorder for borderline patients other than PTSD.

MOOD DISORDERS OVER 16 YEARS
OF PROSPECTIVE FOLLOW-UP

Almost 90% of borderline patients meeting criteria for major depression at baseline experienced a two-year remission by the time of the 16-year follow-up (Zanarini, Hörz-Sagstetter, Frankenburg, Reich, & Fitzmaurice, manuscript under review). Recurrences were about as common (80% for those with remitted major depression). New onsets of major depression were also very common (93% for those without major depression during their index admission), while new onsets of bipolar disorder (mostly bipolar II disorder) occurred in 15% of patients with BPD who had no history of bipolarity at study entry. Taken together, the results of this study suggest that major depression is not a chronic disorder for the majority of borderline patients with co-occurring major depression, but rather is a remitting-recurring disorder. They also suggest an increasing rate of co-occurring bipolar disorder.

In sum, the frequency with which borderline patients meet criteria for other disorders, particularly Axis I disorders, has led to BPD being either thought of as a sub-threshold version of some other disorder or spectrum of disorder, or its very validity being questioned. Yet comorbidity is often encountered in other psychiatric disorders as well as medical disorders. The concept of complex comorbidity, which is now being used by others (Ha, Balderas, Zanarini, Oldham, & Sharp, 2014), is a clinically useful way of using this pattern as a marker for the disorder, which has both affective and impulsive features itself.

14

Mental Health Treatment over Time

Many mental health professionals, as mentioned before in this book, avoid treating those with BPD. This may be due to the physically self-destructive behaviors common among borderline patients (i.e., self-mutilation, suicide gestures and attempts), which can engender fears of being judged negatively by one's colleagues as well as fears of being sued for malpractice. It may also be due to the interpersonal challenges that arise in treating those with BPD, which can engender powerful countertransference feelings. In addition, until relatively recently, there were no evidence-based treatments for BPD. Thus, clinicians may have avoided treating borderline patients because they did not feel sufficiently skilled to handle or help them.

However, there are now five comprehensive forms of psychotherapy that have been found to be superior to treatment as usual or another manualized treatment in reducing the symptoms of BPD. These manual-based psychotherapies are: dialectical behavioral therapy (DBT) (Linehan et al., 1991), mentalization-based treatment (MBT) (Bateman &

Fonagy, 1999), schema-focused therapy (SFT) (Giesen-Bloo et al., 2006), transference-focused psychotherapy (TFP) (Clarkin et al., 2007), and general psychiatric management (GPM) (McMain et al., 2009).

In addition, there are a number of adjunctive group therapies for BPD—the most developed of these being systems training for emotional predictability and problem solving (STEPPS) (Blum et al., 2008). The results of these trials suggest that psychodynamic therapies (MBT and TFP), cognitive behavioral treatments (DBT, SFT, and STEPPS), and therapies that are a combination of both approaches (GPM) are effective in the treatment of BPD.

In addition, psychotropic medications have been found to "take the edge off" BPD symptoms. Before 1995, only four well-designed, double-blind pharmacotherapy studies had been conducted (Cowdry & Gardner, 1988; Salzman et al., 1995; Soloff et al., 1989; Soloff et al., 1993). Since then, the results of 17 double-blind, placebo, or comparator-controlled trials have been published (Black et al., 2014; Bogenschutz & Nurnberg, 2004; Frankenburg & Zanarini, 2002; Hollander et al., 2001; Hollander, Swann, Coccaro, Jiang, & Smith, 2005; Loew et al., 2006; Nickel et al., 2004; Nickel et al., 2005; Rinne, van den Brink, Wouters, & van Dyck, 2002; Schulz, Camlin, Berry, & Friedman, 1999; Schulz et al., 2008; Soler et al., 2005; Tritt et al., 2005; Zanarini & Frankenburg, 2001b; Zanarini & Frankenburg, 2003; Zanarini, Frankenburg, & Parachini, 2004; Zanarini, Schulz, et al., 2011). Taken together, the results of these studies suggest that second-generation antipsychotics, mood stabilizers, and antidepressants all have a modest effect on the severity of borderline psychopathology, but none are curative.

LIFETIME HISTORIES OF PSYCHIATRIC TREATMENT REPORTED DURING INDEX ADMISSION

Given this background, what is the pattern of mental health treatment over time found in the MSAD study? Table 14.1 shows the percentages of borderline patients and Axis II comparison subjects who reported a lifetime

TABLE 14.1   PERCENTAGE OF BORDERLINE PATIENTS AND AXIS II
COMPARISON SUBJECTS WITH LIFETIME HISTORY OF 14 TREATMENT
MODALITIES AT STUDY ENTRY

	BPD %	OPD %
Individual Therapy*	96.2	86.1
Intensive Psychotherapy* (= >2 sessions per week)	36.2	19.4
Group Therapy*	36.2	18.1
Couples/Family Therapy	38.6	29.2
Self-Help Group(s)*	51.0	31.9
Day Treatment*	42.4	19.4
Residential Treatment*	36.9	9.7
Day and/or Residential Treatment*	54.8	23.6
Any Psychiatric Hospitalization*	78.6	50.0
Multiple Hospitalizations*	60.3	20.8
Any Standing Medication*	84.1	61.1
Polypharmacy*	65.5	25.0
Intensive Polypharmacy* (= >3 standing medications)	45.5	12.5
ECT Treatments	6.9	5.6

*Borderline patients (BPD) had significantly higher prevalence rates than Axis II
comparison subjects (OPD).

history of each treatment modality at study entry (Zanarini, Frankenburg,
Khera, et al., 2001). This material was briefly covered in Chapter 4, but a
more careful review of the treatment received before study entrance seems
warranted.

As can be seen, all forms of treatment were common in the histories of
our borderline patients except for electroconvulsive therapy (ECT). In addition, a significantly higher percentage of borderline patients than Axis
II comparison subjects reported participating in each of these treatment
modalities except for couples/family therapy and ECT.

Table 14.2 details the average ages for both patient groups at first entering each treatment modality. As can be seen, borderline patients, on
average, entered most forms of treatment between their late teens and

TABLE 14.2   AGE OF FIRST USE OF TREATMENT MODALITY

	BPD Mean Age	OPD Mean Age
Age at First Individual Therapy*	18.0	22.4
Age at First Group Therapy	22.9	23.3
Age at First Couples/Family Therapy	18.5	20.8
Age at First Self-Help Group(s)	21.5	22.0
Age at First Day Treatment	25.8	26.0
Age at First Residential Treatment	23.6	24.4
Age at First Psychiatric Hospitalization	21.2	24.3
Age at First Standing Medications*	21.6	26.4
Age at First ECT	28.2	37.5

*Borderline patients (BPD) had significantly lower age than Axis II comparison subjects OPD).

mid-twenties. As can also be seen, they were significantly younger than Axis II controls when first entering individual therapy and starting to take standing medications.

TREATMENT OVER SIX YEARS OF PROSPECTIVE FOLLOW-UP

We also studied rates of mental health utilization over the first six years of follow-up (Zanarini, Frankenburg, Hennen, & Silk, 2004). Only 33% of borderline patients were hospitalized during the final two years of the six-year follow-up, a substantial decline from the 79% who had prior hospitalizations at baseline. Much the same pattern emerged for day and/or residential treatment (from 55% to 22%). In contrast, about three-quarters of borderline patients were still in psychotherapy and taking psychotropic medications after six years of follow-up. Additionally, over 70% of border-line patients participating in these outpatient modalities did so for at least 75% of each follow-up period. While rates of intensive psychotherapy declined significantly over time (from 36% to 16%), rates of intensive polypharmacy remained relatively stable over time, with about 40% of borderline patients taking three or more concurrent standing medications during each follow-up period, about 20% taking four or more, and about 10% taking five or more.

We also assessed the treatment received by remitted (about 70%) and non-remitted (about 30%) borderline patients over six years of prospective follow-up. (See Table 14.3.)

We studied four categories of treatment: any outpatient treatment, multiple forms of outpatient treatment, any more-intensive treatment (i.e., day treatment, residential treatment, and psychiatric hospitalizations), and multiple forms of more-intensive treatment. A significantly lower percentage of remitted than non-remitted borderline patients used treatment

TABLE 14.3   PSYCHIATRIC TREATMENT REPORTED BY REMITTED
AND NON-REMITTED BORDERLINE PATIENTS OVER SIX YEARS
OF PROSPECTIVE FOLLOW-UP

Treatment Modality	Remitted Borderline Patients		Non-remitted Borderline Patients	
	BL	6 Yr FU	BL	6 Yr FU
Any Outpatient treatment (individual therapy, standing medication, group therapy, couples/family therapy, self-help group)*	97.0	84.0	100.0	100.0
Multiple Forms of Outpatient Treatment*	91.1	62.0	93.2	90.6
Any More Intensive Treatment (day treatment, residential care, inpatient hospitalization)*	78.2	23.5	89.8	76.6
Multiple Forms of More Intensive Treatment*	49.0	11.5	61.4	46.9

*Each modality was significantly more common among non-remitted than remitted borderline patients. Significant decline for each modality for both study groups.

in each of the four categories studied. However, the prevalence of these categories of treatment declined significantly for those in both groups.

Remitted borderline patients used any outpatient treatment less than non-remitted patients at six-year follow-up, but the percentages were not as disparate (84% vs. 100%) as they were for multiple forms of outpatient treatment (62% vs. 91%). The same pattern was found for any more-intensive treatment (24% vs. 77%) and multiple forms of more-intensive treatment (12% vs. 47%).

The most important take-home messages from these findings are that the majority of borderline patients continue to use outpatient treatment in a sustained manner through six years of follow-up. However, only a declining minority use more restrictive and costly forms of treatment—which makes clinical sense, as less-symptomatic borderline patients would probably use less treatment, particularly more intensive forms of treatment.

TREATMENT OVER 10 YEARS OF PROSPECTIVE FOLLOW-UP

In addition, we studied time-to-cessation and time-to-resumption for three key treatment modalities over ten years of prospective follow-up: individual therapy, standing medications, and psychiatric hospitalizations (Hörz, Zanarini, Frankenburg, Reich, & Fitzmaurice, 2010). In terms of time-to-cessation and resumption, 52% of patients with BPD stopped individual therapy and 44% stopped taking standing medications for a period of two years or more (at least one follow-up period). However, 85% of those who had stopped psychotherapy resumed it, and 67% of those who stopped taking medications later resumed taking them. In contrast, 88% had no hospitalizations for at least two years, but almost half of these patients were subsequently rehospitalized.

While four additional years of follow-up were studied and a different way to view the data was used (time-to-event rather than prevalence rates), the conclusions were very similar to those after six years of follow-up. More specifically, these results suggest that patients with BPD tend to use outpatient treatment without interruption over prolonged periods of time. They also suggest that inpatient treatment is used far more intermittently and by only a relative small minority of those with BPD.

TREATMENT OVER 16 YEARS OF PROSPECTIVE FOLLOW-UP

We also studied the prevalence rates of 16 forms of treatment over 16 years of prospective follow-up (Zanarini, Frankenburg, Reich, Conkey, & Fitzmaurice, 2015). Patients with BPD were not significantly more likely to report being in individual therapy, intensive individual therapy, or couples/family therapy than those with other Axis II disorders. However, they were significantly more likely to report being in group therapy and self-help groups. They were also significantly more likely to report taking any standing medication, all forms of polypharmacy studied (2–5 standing medications), and all forms of more intensive treatment studied except ECT (day treatment, residential treatment, psychiatric hospitalizations, multiple psychiatric hospitalizations, and 30 days or more of hospitalization).

During the first eight years of follow-up (0–8 years), reported rates of all forms of treatment were found to decline significantly for those in both study groups, except taking four or five or more concurrent medications and ECT. Conversely, during the last eight years of follow-up (8–16 years), reported rates of almost all forms of treatment remained relatively flat or stable over time for both study groups; the only exception was the rate of 30 days or more of psychiatric hospitalization, which continued to decline significantly for those in both study groups.

Here we get a clear picture of the tendency of borderline patients to continue in many treatment modalities over a sustained period of time, with decline in prevalence rates occurring in the first eight years of follow-up and then a pattern of stable treatment-use appearing.

SPECIFIC CLASSES AND TYPES
OF PSYCHOTROPIC MEDICATION OVER 16 YEARS
OF PROSPECTIVE FOLLOW-UP

We also studied the rates of various types of psychotropic medication over
16 years of prospective follow-up (Zanarini, Frankenburg, Reich, Harned,
& Fitzmaurice, 2015). It was found that a significantly higher percentage
of borderline patients than Axis II comparison subjects reported taking
an antidepressant, an anxiolytic, an antipsychotic, and a mood stabilizer
over time. Specifically, the reported rates of antidepressants were approximately 30% higher for borderline patients than for Axis II comparison
subjects; the reported rates of anxiolytics and antipsychotics were 2.6
times higher, while the reported rates of mood stabilizers were approximately 3 times higher.

The rates for both study groups reporting taking an antidepressant
and an anxiolytic declined significantly from baseline to eight-year
follow-up, but not from eight-year follow-up to 16-year follow-up. The
rates of antipsychotics and mood stabilizers did not decline significantly in either eight-year-long follow-up time period for those in either
study group.

In terms of the four more specific types of antidepressants, a significantly higher percentage of borderline patients than Axis II comparison
subjects reported taking a selective serotonin reuptake inhibitor (SSRI)
and an atypical antidepressant, but not a tricyclic or a monoamine oxidase
(MAO) inhibitor. Both types of anxiolytics studied—benzodiazepines and
non-benzodiazepines—were reported by a significantly higher percentage
of borderline patients than by Axis II comparison subjects. In terms of
antipsychotics, a significantly higher percentage of borderline patients reported taking a conventional but not an atypical antipsychotic. Both types
of mood stabilizer studied—anticonvulsants and lithium—were reported
by a significantly higher percentage of borderline patients than by Axis II
comparison subjects

Over time, both study groups reported a significantly declining rate
of taking an SSRI, a tricyclic, an MAO inhibitor, a benzodiazepine, and

lithium from baseline to eight-year follow-up, but not eight-year follow-up to 16-year follow-up. Those in both study groups reported a significantly declining rate of taking a non-benzodiazepine anxiolytic and a conventional antipsychotic as well as a significantly increasing rate of taking an atypical antipsychotic at both follow-up time periods. Only the reported rates of taking an atypical antidepressant and an anticonvulsant remained stable over time for those in both study groups (i.e., did not decline significantly at either follow-up time period).

RESULTS FROM THE CLPS STUDY

Psychiatric treatment was assessed at baseline and at three-year follow-up. At baseline, patients with BPD were significantly more likely than depressed patients to have received every type of psychosocial treatment studied except self-help groups (i.e., individual, group, and family/couples therapy; day treatment, psychiatric hospitalization, and halfway house residence [Bender et al., 2001]). Patients with BPD were also more likely to have used antianxiety, antidepressant, antipsychotic medications, and mood stabilizers. In addition, patients with BPD had received greater amounts of treatment, except for family/couples therapy and self-help, than the depressed patients and those with other forms of personality disorder.

At three-year follow-up, patients with BPD were significantly more likely than those with major depressive disorder to use all types of treatment studied (i.e., individual therapy, medications, emergency department visits, and hospitalizations). In addition, borderline patients continued using high-intensity, low-duration treatments throughout the study period, albeit at low rates of prevalence, while individual psychotherapy attendance declined significantly after one year.

These findings are quite different than those in MSAD. It may be due to the fact that most CLPS participants were outpatients at study entrance. They were also about a decade older than MSAD participants.

MOST COMMON TREATMENT MODALITIES

Two of these modalities are outpatient treatments (therapy and medication). The third is more intensive (psychiatric hospitalizations).

Psychotherapy

Most patients in the study were treated in the community by psychologists or social workers for psychotherapy and by psychiatrists or primary care physicians for medication. Almost none were ever in an evidence-based treatment for BPD, because most of these treatments were introduced after the study had been going on for a number of years and there was a lack of availability of qualified treaters, even to this day.

Most of these therapies seemed to be a combination of supportive and cognitive behavioral approaches. However, it is not clear what these therapies focused on. It may initially have been on symptom amelioration. However, it would be hoped that these treatments then focused on the patients' retaining their functioning in the social and vocational realms; recapturing the achievements in these areas that they have lost; or attaining them for the first time. And yet the high rates of patients, particularly those who have not recovered, receiving disability payments suggest that this is not so. It may be that such a patient is so impaired that this federal benefit is the only source of income on which she can depend. It may also be that her distress was intolerable to her and her therapist, who mistook inner pain for impairment.

Psychotropic Medication

Many borderline patients in the study have been tried on a wide variety of medications. In our experience, they are often on three or more standing medications at any one time. Not only is this expensive, but it is not clear how effective this approach is, as the only study that compared monotherapy to polypharmacy in a sample of borderline patients found that these approaches were equally efficacious (Zanarini, Frankenburg, &

Parachini, 2004). In addition, there are serious side effects to most psychiatric medications, particularly weight gain. This is a serious problem for a substantial percentage of the borderline patients in the study, as their obesity or near-obesity may interfere with their social life, and may, over the long run, be deleterious to their physical health as well. (See Chapter 15 for more details.) Another consideration is that having ready access to a number of different medications can result in more lethal suicide attempts should the decision be made, either in a planned or impulsive manner, to ingest a large and indiscriminant quantity of these medications.

Psychiatric Hospitalizations

Sometimes borderline patients are so depressed, suicidal, or out of control that they need to be hospitalized. Very few treaters still believe that a hospitalization should be prolonged or that it constitutes a "growth" experience. Rather, due to economic pressures, treaters have come to see hospitalizations as brief experiences whose main purpose is to stabilize the functioning of a borderline patient. Now, when borderline patients say they feel much better the day after being admitted for cutting themselves, they are likely to be believed. In most cases, this works out well, but in some cases, such a rapid move toward discharge can have tragic consequences.

Brief hospitalizations promise less and typically lead to less regression. However, there are times when a borderline patient may need to stay in the hospital for weeks or even months at a time. This is so when they are deeply and perhaps psychotically depressed. It may also be so when they have managed to alienate everyone in their life to the extent that they have no meaningful relationships and suicide is a real option for them, as they no longer have any social supports.

Regardless of the length of the hospitalization, borderline patients often resist being discharged. Sometimes they are able to discuss this with staff, and sometimes they act out to stay in. Often these end-stage regressions can be avoided by anticipating them. If their fear and anger at being discharged are predicted and discussed throughout their inpatient stay, they may be able to have a cognitive map of what is going on and state their objections in a straightforward manner, or simply go ahead with the discharge without resorting to regressive delaying tactics. These tactics, such as begging to stay or losing control and being put in a quiet room, are time-consuming and stressful for all involved. They may also lead to feelings of shame and defeat for the borderline patient who feels as if his pain and desperation are being downplayed or ignored.

15

Physical Health and Medical Treatment

M any clinicians with limited experience working with patients with BPD tend to think of them as they were when the clinicians were trainees—young and physically healthy. However, patients with BPD do grow older, and some have better physical health than others.

CHRONIC MEDICAL CONDITIONS, POOR HEALTH-RELATED LIFESTYLE CHOICES, AND COSTLY FORMS OF MEDICAL CARE: CROSS-SECTIONAL RESULTS AT SIX-YEAR FOLLOW-UP

We began to study their physical health at six-year follow-up using an interview designed specifically for this project (Frankenburg & Zanarini, 2004b). We first examined the physical health, health-related life style choices, and use of medical treatment of 200 ever-remitted borderline patients and 64 never-remitted borderline patients at six-year follow-up, who, on average, were then in their early thirties.

Remitted borderline patients were found to be significantly less likely than non-remitted borderline patients to have a history of a "syndrome-like" condition (i.e., chronic fatigue, fibromyalgia, or temporomandibular joint [TMJ] syndrome) (25% vs. 42%), or to have a history of obesity (24% vs. 41%), osteoarthritis (8% vs. 17%), diabetes (2% vs, 11%), hypertension (5% vs. 13%), back pain (39% vs, 63%), or urinary incontinence (5% vs, 19%). They were also found to be significantly less likely to report pack-per-day smoking (41% vs. 61%), daily consumption of alcohol (25% vs. 44%), lack of regular exercise (47% vs. 69%), daily use of sleep medications (22% vs. 63%), and sustained use of pain medications (27% vs. 41%). In addition, remitted borderline patients were significantly less likely than non-remitted borderline patients to have had at least one medically-related emergency room visit (51% vs. 80%) and/or medical hospitalization (18% vs. 41%) (both of which did not include pregnancy-related visits or hospitalizations). Ever-remitted borderline patients were also found to be significantly less likely than those who never-remitted to have a history of multiple medical conditions (26% vs. 58%) as well as both a medically-related ER visit and a medical hospitalization (17% vs. 42%).

It is important to note that this pattern of poor health (among both groups of borderline patients to some extent) did not occur as a result of a lack of medical care. More specifically, the majority of those in both patient groups had an annual physical, saw their primary care physician or a specialist at least once in the two-year period covered by the interview, and had regular dental care. Only about 20% of each group had any trouble accessing medical care or paying for it. However, non-remitted borderline patients were significantly more likely than remitted borderline patients to have quit work or lost a job because of poor health.

CHRONIC MEDICAL CONDITIONS, POOR HEALTH-
RELATED LIFESTYLE CHOICES, AND COSTLY
FORMS OF MEDICAL CARE: LONGITUDINAL
RESULTS FROM SIX- TO 16-YEAR FOLLOW-UP

We later studied chronic medical conditions, health-related life style choices, and costly forms of medical care in this same sample of borderline patients followed for 10 years (from 6-year follow-up to 16-year follow-up) (Keuroghlian, Frankenburg, & Zanarini, 2013). We compared those who had recovered (concurrent symptomatic remission and good social and good full-time vocational functioning) to those who had not recovered. Ever-recovered borderline patients were significantly less likely than never-recovered borderline patients to have a medical syndrome, obesity, osteoarthritis, diabetes, urinary incontinence, or multiple medical conditions. They were also significantly less likely to report pack-per-day smoking, weekly alcohol use, no regular exercise, daily sleep medication use, or pain medication use. In addition, ever-recovered borderline patients were significantly less likely than never-recovered borderline patients to undergo a medical emergency room visit, medical hospitalization, X-ray, CT scan, or MRI scan.

OBESITY AND OBESITY-RELATED CONDITIONS

We also studied the prevalence, risk factors, and consequences for obesity in borderline patients in general at six-year follow-up (Frankenburg & Zanarini, 2006). Body mass index (BMI) was computed for each subject using their measured height and weight from their index admission and their self-reported height and weight at six-year follow-up. BMI was calculated by dividing the weight in kilograms by the square of the height in meters. Twenty-eight percent of these 264 borderline patients had a BMI of 30 or greater. Six years earlier, at baseline, only 17% of these 264 borderline patients had been obese. Of the 74 obese patients, 36% were extremely or morbidly obese, which is typically defined as having a BMI of at least 40.

Four significant risk factors for obesity in these borderline patients were found: chronic PTSD, lack of exercise, a family history of obesity, and a recent history of aggressive psychotropic polypharmacy (three or more standing psychiatric medications). A lack of exercise, a family history of obesity, and being treated with aggressive polypharmacy are risk factors for obesity in many patient populations. However, the addition of chronic PTSD suggests that exposure to trauma in childhood and/or adulthood joins these other factors in those with BPD to heighten the risk of obesity. The reason for this is unclear. It may be that they are too frightened or despondent to exercise regularly. It may also be that they are treated more aggressively with psychotropic medications than other patients with BPD. In addition, they may share a genetic risk for weight gain with their close family members and/or have grown up in an environment where being obese was neither unusual nor stigmatized.

In terms of health consequences, they were significantly more likely than the non-obese borderline patients to report suffering from nine disorders. These disorders are: diabetes, hypertension, osteoarthritis, chronic back pain, carpal tunnel syndrome, urinary incontinence, gastroesophageal reflux disorder (GERD), gallstones, and asthma. While these co-occurring disorders are common among obese populations in general, this study highlighted that obesity hastened the onset of these disorders in those with BPD and obesity.

We next examined the relationship between cumulative body mass index (CBMI) and symptomatic, psychosocial, and medical outcomes in patients with BPD (Frankenburg & Zanarini, 2011). Two hundred female borderline patients were weighed and measured during their index admission. They were subsequently interviewed at six-, eight-, and 10-year intervals. Over 10 years of prospective follow-up, increases in cumulative BMI were significantly associated with self-mutilation and dissociation (but not suicide attempts). Increases in cumulative BMI were also significantly associated with having no life partner, a poor work or school history, being on disability, being rated with a GAF score in the fair or poor range, and having a low income. In addition, increases in BMI were related to having two or more additional medical conditions and using costly forms of health care. Taken together, increases in cumulative BMI may be a marker for adverse symptomatic, functional, and medical outcomes in patients with BPD.

SLEEP DISTURBANCES

Sleep disturbance is a common, yet poorly understood, phenomenon in BPD. We examined the use of sedative-hypnotic medication in those with BPD over six years of follow-up (6–10-year follow-up) (Plante, Zanarini, Frankenburg, & Fitzmaurice, 2009). In comparison to other personality disorder (OPD) comparison subjects, a significantly higher percentage of BPD subjects than OPD subjects used both as needed (prn) and standing medications to help them sleep. Specifically, over the course of the study, BPD subjects were approximately four times more likely to have used prn and standing sleep medications. When adjusted for differences in depression, anxiety, and age among BPD and OPD subjects, BPD subjects were approximately three times more likely to have used prn and standing sleeping medications. These results indicate that sedative-hypnotic use is greater among BPD than among OPD subjects. They also confirm clinical observations that subjective sleep disturbance is a significant problem in BPD.

As noted, patients with BPD frequently experience sleep disturbance. However, the role of sleep quality in the course of BPD is unknown. We wanted to begin to fill that gap in knowledge by evaluating the cross-sectional association between sleep quality and recovery status (symptomatic remission plus good concurrent psychosocial functioning) in a well-characterized cohort of patients with BPD (Plante, Frankenburg, Fitzmaurice, & Zanarini, 2013a).

Accordingly, 223 patients with BPD were administered the Pittsburgh Sleep Quality Index (PSQI) as part of the 16-year follow-up wave (Carpenter & Andrykowski, 1998). This questionnaire consists of directed response and Likert-scale (4-point) questions regarding seven component areas: sleep quality, latency, duration, efficiency, disturbance, use of sleeping medications, and daytime dysfunction. Responses in each category are scored to range from 0–3, and the global score equals the sum of the seven components (maximum score, 21), with higher scores indicating greater sleep disturbance.

Sleep quality was compared between recovered (N = 105) and non-recovered (N = 118) BPD participants, including adjustments for age, sex, depression, anxiety, and primary sleep disorders. Non-recovered BPD patients had significantly worse sleep quality than recovered BPD participants, as measured by the global PSQI score. In addition, non-recovered BPD participants had longer sleep-onset latency (adjusted means 39 vs. 28 minutes), as well as increased odds of using sleeping medication and experiencing daytime dysfunction as a result of their sleep disturbance.

These results demonstrate an association between subjective sleep disturbance and recovery status among BPD patients. Further research is indicated to evaluate the mechanisms underlying sleep disturbance in BPD, and to see whether treatment of sleep complaints improves the symptomatic and psychosocial course of the disorder.

Because dysfunctional beliefs and attitudes are common among patients with insomnia, we wanted to evaluate the association between maladaptive sleep-related cognitions and recovery status in patients with BPD (Plante, Frankenburg, Fitzmaurice, & Zanarini, 2013b). Two hundred and twenty-three BPD patients were administered the Dysfunctional Beliefs and Attitudes about Sleep questionnaire (DBAS-16) (Morin, Vallières, & Ivers, 2007) as part of the 16-year follow-up wave.

Questions on the DBAS-16 fall into one of four thematic subscale/factors: (1) perceived consequences of insomnia (Consequence), (2) worry/helplessness about insomnia (Worry/Helplessness), (3) expectations about sleep (Expectations), and (4) attitudes about sleep medications (Medication). Five questions compose the Consequence factor, each related broadly to the subject's perception of how insomnia affects energy, mood, and overall functioning. The Worry/Helplessness subscale comprises six questions, focused on perceptions and beliefs about how worried a subject may be about the unpredictable nature of his/her sleep, and how it may affect their vitality and health. The Expectations factor is composed of two questions, regarding the belief that one cannot function without eight hours of sleep, and that napping or sleeping in the next day is necessary to catch up on sleep if preceded by a night of insomnia. Finally, the Medication subscale is comprised of three questions, which query the participant regarding beliefs that insomnia is essentially the result of a chemical imbalance and can only be managed by medications. The average of all 16 questions forms the overall DBAS-16 score, with higher scores indicating a greater degree of maladaptive sleep-related cognitions.

Maladaptive sleep cognitions were compared between recovered (N = 105) and non-recovered (N = 118) BPD participants, in analyses that adjusted for age, sex, depression, anxiety, and primary sleep disorders. Results demonstrated that non-recovered BPD patients had significantly more severe maladaptive sleep-related cognitions as measured by the overall DBAS-16 score. These results demonstrate an association between dysfunctional beliefs and attitudes about sleep and recovery status among BPD patients. Further research is warranted to evaluate treatments targeted towards maladaptive sleep-related cognitions, and their subsequent effects on the course of BPD.

PHYSICAL PAIN

Patients with BPD frequently present to primary care physicians and specialists with pain problems. We wanted to (1) examine the prevalence of pain symptoms in patients with a diagnosis of BPD compared with a diagnosis of another personality disorder, and (2) identify the factors that predict the pain experienced in patients with BPD (Biskin, Frankenburg, Fitzmaurice, & Zanarini, 2014). Ratings of pain were assessed 16 years after baseline diagnosis and compared between diagnostic groups.

Patients with BPD are more likely to experience pain and rate their pain as more severe than patients with other personality disorders. In multivariable models, there were three significant predictors of severity of pain among patients with BPD: older age, the presence of major depressive disorder, and the severity of childhood abuse other than sexual abuse (emotional, verbal, and physical abuse).

Patients with BPD reported significant pain, which interferes with their lives. A focus on the management of medical and psychiatric comorbidities may improve their long-term functioning.

We also focused on opioid use to treat physical pain over 10 years of prospective follow-up (from 6–16-year follow-up) (Frankenburg, Fitzmaurice, & Zanarini, 2014). It was found that borderline patients were significantly more likely to report the use of prescription opioid medication over time than Axis II comparison subjects (26% vs. 16% at 16-year follow-up). The best predictors of opioid use among borderline patients were the time-varying presence of back pain, fibromyalgia, and osteoarthritis, as well as a baseline (but not follow-up) history of drug abuse. The sustained use of prescription opioids is common among and discriminating for patients with BPD. The results also suggest that these borderline patients may be particularly sensitive to physical pain—mirroring their well-known heightened sensitivity to emotional pain.

IRRITABLE BOWEL SYNDROME

We also examined rates of irritable bowel syndrome (IBS) over 10 years of prospective follow-up among recovered and non-recovered patients with BPD (Niesten, Karan, Frankenburg, Fitzmaurice, & Zanarini, 2014). Subsequently, risk factors for IBS were examined in female BPD patients. As part of MSAD, 264 BPD patients were assessed at baseline, and their medical conditions and time-varying predictors of IBS were assessed over five waves of follow-up (from 6-year follow-up to 16-year follow-up). Semi-structured interviews were used to assess both our IBS outcome variable and our baseline and time-varying predictor variables. Rates of IBS were not significantly different between recovered and non-recovered borderline patients when men and women were considered together and when men were considered alone. However, a significant difference in IBS rates was found between recovered and non-recovered female BPD patients, with the latter reporting significantly higher rates. The rates of IBS in women with BPD were found to be significantly predicted by a family history of IBS and a childhood history of verbal, emotional, and/ or physical abuse. The results of this study suggest that both biological/ social learning factors and childhood adversity may be risk factors for IBS in women with BPD.

16

Adult Victimization over Time

erman (1986; Herman & van der Kolk, 1987) was the first to suggest that borderline patients have elevated rates of physical assault and/or rape as adults and to note that such experiences might be associated with traumatic childhood events. Although ten studies have since confirmed that a high percentage of borderline patients, particularly inpatients, report having experienced physical and/or sexual abuse as children (see Chapter 2), a study we conducted using our baseline sample was the first to have explicitly examined the prevalence of experiences of violence in the lives of adult borderline patients (Zanarini et al., 1999). It was also the first to have examined their association with childhood trauma and other risk factors.

BASELINE FINDINGS

We found that 46% of borderline patients reported having been a victim of violence since the age of 18, our cutoff age for being an adult. In terms of specific forms of violence, 33% of our borderline patients reported having had a physically abusive partner, 31% reported that they had been raped, 21% reported that they had been raped by a known perpetrator, and 11% reported a history of multiple rapes. In addition, 19% of the borderline patients in the study reported both having had a physically abusive partner and having been raped.

It was also found that borderline patients were significantly more likely than Axis II comparison subjects to report having had a physically abusive partner, having been raped, having been raped by a known perpetrator, having been raped multiple times, and having both been physically assaulted by a partner and raped. Female borderline patients were significantly more likely than male borderline patients to have been physically and/or sexually assaulted as adults (50% vs. 26%). However, a significantly higher percentage of borderline patients of both genders reported experiences of adult violence than comparison subjects of the same gender. In addition, four risk factors were found to significantly predict whether borderline patients had an adult history of being a victim of violence: female gender, a SUD that began before the age of 18, childhood sexual abuse, and emotional withdrawal by a caretaker (which we classified as a form of neglect).

Taken together, these results suggest that childhood experiences of both reported abuse and neglect are risk factors for experiences of violence in adulthood. It may be that borderline patients are primed to be treated violently due to their childhood history of sexual abuse. It may also be that they do not expect others around them to be emotionally available enough to protect them or to come to their aid when their physical integrity is being threatened. In addition, having a juvenile history of substance abuse that continued into adulthood may decrease their inhibitions and impair their judgement, making it difficult to perceive the danger in certain situations or relationships.

FINDINGS OVER SIX YEARS OF PROSPECTIVE FOLLOW-UP

We also studied these forms of adult violence over six years of prospective follow-up. In addition, we studied the course of being verbally and emotionally abused as an adult (i.e., being 18 or older) (Zanarini, Frankenburg, Reich, Hennen, & Silk, 2005). It was found that each of these types of abuse was reported by a significantly higher percentage of borderline patients than Axis II comparison subjects over time. The rates of all four forms of reported abuse declined significantly over time for all subjects considered together. For borderline patients, the decline from baseline to six-year follow-up was as follows: verbal abuse (76% vs. 33%), emotional abuse (71% vs. 37%), physical abuse (33% vs. 12%), and sexual abuse (31% vs. 7%). In addition, verbal, emotional, and physical abuse in adulthood, but not sexual abuse, was a significant predictor of a slower time-to-remission of BPD as well as a diminished likelihood of attaining remission from BPD.

The nature of the relationship between these adult experiences and remission from BPD is unknown. It may be that borderline patients who have had abusive relationships or experiences in adulthood have less emotional energy to focus on getting well and attaining a remission of BPD. It may also be that adult experiences of abuse are markers for a more chronic type of borderline psychopathology.

FINDINGS OVER 10 YEARS OF PROSPECTIVE FOLLOW-UP

We also conducted a study of this topic after 10 years of prospective follow-up (McGowan, King, Frankenburg, Fitzmaurice, & Zanarini, 2012). Over time, it was found that the rates of all four types of abuse declined significantly for borderline patients, although remaining significantly higher for borderline patients than for Axis II comparison subjects. More specifically, at 10-year follow-up, 29% of borderline patients reported being verbally abused, 29% reported being emotionally abused, 6% reported being physically abused or assaulted, and 4% reported being sexually abused or raped. For borderline patients who reported these experiences at baseline, rates of cessation (for two years or more) were high for all types of abuse (>90%). However, recurrences and new onsets of verbal and emotional abuse were relatively common (>60%). Contrastingly, they were relatively uncommon for physical and sexual abuse (<30%), suggesting that verbal and emotional abuse represent more stable forms of abuse, or forms of abuse that are more socially acceptable to speak about.

The results of all of these studies suggest that being a victim of adult violence is common in the lives of borderline patients, particularly women with BPD. They also suggest significantly declining rates over extended periods of time, and even very high rates of actual cessation for all four forms of being abused as an adult. However, the rates of subsequent recurrences and new onsets of verbal and emotional abuse were high for borderline patients, while the rates of physical and sexual abuse were substantially lower.

These results may have implications for treatment. More specifically, it might be helpful if clinicians are aware of the fluidity of adult experiences of abuse, particularly concerning recurrences and new onsets. They could be better prepared to help their borderline patients anticipate potential dangers. They could also be better prepared to help a person with BPD who has been victimized by someone whom she probably knows.

It should be noted that each type of abuse at each time period was only counted if a patient was able to provide a convincing example of that type of abuse. For example, being told that he was stupid, ugly, and the cause of all of the family's problems was counted as verbal abuse. However, having someone suggest that getting a job might be helpful was not counted, even if it was reported as an example of such abuse.

17

Sexual Issues over Time

We studied two types of sexual issues among borderline patients and Axis II comparison subjects over time. The first issue was "sexual relationship difficulties," which we defined as avoiding sex for fear of becoming symptomatic or becoming symptomatic after having sex. The second area of study related to sexuality or intimacy was sexual orientation and gender of relationship choice.

SEXUAL RELATIONSHIP DIFFICULTIES OVER SIX YEARS OF PROSPECTIVE FOLLOW-UP

We first studied sexual relationship difficulties after six years of prospective follow-up (Zanarini, Parachini, et al., 2003). Sexual relationship difficulties were found to be significantly more common among borderline patients than among Axis II comparison subjects (61% vs. 19%). Sexual relationship difficulties were also found to be significantly more common

among women than men with BPD (65% vs. 43%). Rates of sexual relationship difficulties declined for both borderline patients and Axis II
comparison subjects over time, but the changes were more pronounced
for borderline patients, particularly male borderline patients. In addition, three significant predictors of sexual relationship difficulties among
borderline patients emerged: female gender, reported childhood history
of sexual abuse, and adult history of rape. The results of this study suggest
that problematic sexual relationships may be more common among borderline patients than previously recognized.

It is not surprising that both a reported childhood history of sexual
abuse and an adult history of rape were significantly associated with an
adult pattern of sexual relationship difficulties, even after controlling
for gender. One would expect that sexual trauma, whether in childhood and/or adulthood, would predispose many people to avoiding
consensual sexual experiences for fear that they would trigger a recrudescence of trauma-related memories and/or symptoms. The dif-
ferential rates of childhood sexual abuse (46% vs. 67%) and adult rape
histories (14% vs. 36%) reported by men and women, respectively, in
this sample of borderline patients also helps to explain the difference
in rates of sexual relationship difficulties reported by male and female
borderline patients.

Equally important, our findings concerning sexual relationship
difficulties suggest an apparently unrecognized reason for the stormy
relationships with partners or spouses that characterize the personal
lives of many borderline patients. As is well known, many borderline
patients are highly affiliative by nature and often become quite dependent
on those to whom they feel closest (Gunderson & Links, 2008). Their
oscillating pattern of clinging to and fleeing from intimate relationships
is also well known (Gunderson & Links, 2008). Psychodynamic thinkers
have explained this pattern as being due to abandonment fears followed
by fears of engulfment or annihilation (Adler & Buie, 1979). It is equally
likely that borderline patients, like most people, feel a deep need to be
close to their romantic partners or spouses, but that those with prior
experiences of sexual victimization may either avoid such experiences of

intimacy for fear of becoming seriously symptomatic and/or developing serious symptoms as a result of having consensual sex.

Of course, there are other reasons for such sexual relationship difficulties. For example, some borderline patients may have identified with a parent or parents whom they watched avoiding sex or complaining of its disquieting effects after the fact. They may also be involved with a partner or spouse who is not optimally sensitive to their needs in this area.

Whatever the reason or reasons behind such avoidant and/or symptomatic behavior, the results of this study suggest that clinicians could be even more helpful to the borderline patients they treat if they paid more attention to the sexual parameters of their intimate relationships. It is possible that adequately addressing the fears of such borderline patients might help to improve the quality of what may well be their most important adult relationships.

SEXUAL RELATIONSHIP DIFFICULTIES OVER 16 YEARS OF PROSPECTIVE FOLLOW-UP

We also studied this topic after 16 years of prospective follow-up (Karan, Niesten, Frankenburg, Fitzmaurice, & Zanarini, 2016). We compared recovered borderline patients to non-recovered borderline patients. The prevalence of sexual relationship difficulties declined significantly over time for both groups of patients, while remaining significantly more common among non-recovered borderline patients. More specifically, 31% of recovered borderline patients and 52% of non-recovered borderline patients endorsed avoidance of sex at baseline. And 25% of recovered borderline patients and 44% of non-recovered borderline patients endorsed becoming symptomatic after sex at baseline. These rates at 16-year follow-up were 7% versus 25% for avoidance of sex for recovered and non-recovered borderline patients and 7% versus 13% for symptomatic after sex for recovered and non-recovered borderline patients.

We also examined the time course of those who had each of these symptoms at baseline. By 16-year follow-up, over 95% of each group of patients achieved remission for both types of sexual relationship difficulty. Recurrences of avoidance of sex were significantly more common in non-recovered patients than in recovered patients (82% vs. 45%). However, rates of recurrences of becoming symptomatic after sex did not differ significantly between non-recovered and recovered borderline patients (48% vs. 60%). In addition, non-recovered patients had significantly higher rates of new onsets compared to recovered patients for each type of sexual relationship difficulty: avoidance of sex (55% vs. 21%) and symptomatic after sex (55% vs. 28%).

SEXUAL ORIENTATION AND SEXUAL RELATIONSHIP CHOICE

We assessed sexual orientation and gender of relationship choice over 10 years of prospective follow-up for both borderline patients and Axis II comparison subjects (Reich & Zanarini, 2008). Patients with BPD were significantly more likely than Axis II comparison subjects to report homosexual or bisexual orientation and intimate same-sex relationships. There were no significant differences between male and female borderline subjects in prevalence of reported homosexual or bisexual orientation or in prevalence of reported same-sex relationships. Patients with BPD were significantly more likely than Axis II comparison subjects to report changing the gender of intimate partners, but not sexual orientation, at some point during the follow-up period.

We also studied predictors of these two outcomes. A family history of homosexual or bisexual orientation was the only significant predictor of an aggregate outcome variable assessing homosexual/bisexual orientation and/or same sex relationship in borderline subjects. Results of this study suggest that same-gender attraction and/or intimate relationship choice may be an important interpersonal issue for approximately one-third of both men and women with BPD.

Some may see these results as indicative of an identity disturbance in borderline patients. It is equally likely that these results represent a strength for borderline patients. More specifically, they are more willing than others to affiliate with the person who at the moment—man or woman—who can best help them grow and adapt to the changing course of their adult life.

18

Defense Mechanisms over Time

Anna Freud (1937) was one of the first psychoanalysts to carefully describe a series of defense mechanisms that underlay most forms of psychopathology that were identified at that time. "Defense mechanisms" are defined as unconscious ways of handling stress or coping with stress. As the influence of psychoanalysis has waned in the past 20 years, many mental health professionals are unfamiliar with this construct, and some are actively hostile to it. However, some have kept this area of research moving forward. Foremost among these researchers are George Vaillant (1986), J. Christopher Perry (Perry & Cooper, 1986), and Michael Bond (Bond, 1990; Bond, Paris, & Zweig-Frank, 1994).

We have administered Bond's Defense Style Questionnaire (Bond, 1991) at each assessment period from baseline to 16 years after index admission, or nine separate times. We studied 19 specific defenses. These defenses are organized partly by Vaillant's empirically derived hierarchy of defenses (1986): mature, neurotic, and immature defenses. The remaining defenses are organized according to Kernberg's theoretical model of borderline defenses (1967).

Box 18.1 lists these defenses and their level of defensive functioning. It should be noted that Vaillant's immature defenses, which he believes underlie personality disorders, are roughly at the same level as the borderline defenses, which Kernberg believes underlie borderline personality organization, a broad category that encompasses most personality disorders.

It should be noted that we added three items to more fully measure the defense of emotional hypochondriasis that we have described elsewhere (Zanarini & Frankenburg, 1994). These three items ("No matter how often I tell people how miserable I feel, no one really seems to believe me"; "No matter what I say or do, I can't seem to get other people to really understand how much emotional agony I'm in"; "I often act in ways that are self-destructive to get other people to pay attention to the tremendous emotional pain that I'm in") were combined with the three already present to measure the related defense of help-rejecting complaining ("Doctors never really understand what is wrong with me"; "My doctors are not able to help me really get over my problems"; "No matter how much I complain, I never get a satisfactory response").

CROSS-SECTIONAL BASELINE DEFENSES

Using cross-sectional baseline data (Zanarini, Weingeroff, & Frankenburg, 2009), it was found that borderline patients had significantly higher scores than Axis II comparison subjects on one neurotic-level defense (undoing), four immature defenses (acting out, emotional hypochondriasis [i.e., transformation of feelings of sorrow, rage, and terror into unremitting complaints about the lack of understanding that others display], passive aggression, and projection), and two image-distorting/borderline defenses (projective identification and splitting). In contrast, Axis II comparison subjects had significantly higher scores than borderline patients on one mature defense (suppression).

Box 18.1 DEFENSE MECHANISMS STUDIED

Vaillant's Mature Defenses

Altruism
Anticipation
Humor
Sublimation
Suppression

Vaillant's Neurotic Defenses

Isolation
Reaction Formation
Undoing

Vaillant's Immature Defenses

Acting Out
Denial
Emotional Hypochondriasis
Fantasy
Passive Aggression
Projection

Image Distorting or Borderline Defenses

Devaluation
Omnipotence
Primitive Idealization
Projective Identification
Splitting

All four of these immature defenses underlie clinical features (impulsivity, demandingness, masochism, and suspiciousness) that have been found to be extremely common among borderline patients (Zanarini, Gunderson, Frankenburg, & Chauncey, 1990). As we noted before, two image distorting/borderline defenses were found to differentiate borderline patients from Axis II comparison subjects. More specifically, borderline patients had significantly higher mean scores on the defenses of projective identification and splitting than Axis II comparison subjects did.

Of equal importance is that three other image distorting/borderline defenses were not found to differentiate borderline patients from Axis II comparison subjects: devaluation, omnipotence, and primitive idealization. Taken together, these results are consistent with the earlier findings of Perry and Cooper (1986) who found that what they termed "borderline defenses" (projective identification and splitting) were strongly associated with borderline psychopathology, while what they termed "narcissistic defenses" (devaluation, omnipotence, and primitive idealization) were not. This failure to confirm Kernberg's defensive typology may well be due to the broader concept of borderline personality organization that Kernberg espoused; a concept that includes patients with other severe personality disorders as well as BPD.

In addition, three defenses were found in multivariate analyses to be significantly associated with a borderline diagnosis: acting out, emotional hypochondriasis, and undoing (Table 18.1).

TABLE 18.1   MULTIVARIATE DEFENSE MECHANISMS PREDICTIVE OF BORDERLINE DIAGNOSIS AND TIME-TO-RECOVERY

Defense Mechanisms Predictive of Borderline Diagnosis at Study Entry	Defense Mechanisms Predictive of Time-to-Recovery
Acting Out	Acting Out
Emotional Hypochondriasis	Emotional Hypochondriasis
Undoing	Projection
	Humor

This finding makes clinical sense, as impulsivity, demandingness, and making amends are aspects of a pattern that is characteristic of borderline patients. This finding also indicates that the presence of this trio of defenses is a good marker for the borderline diagnosis. This model has both good sensitivity (.95) and positive predictive power (.86).

The results of this study suggest that the defensive profile of borderline patients is distinct from that of patients with other forms of Axis II pathology. They also suggest that the defensive triad of acting out, emotional hypochondriasis, and undoing may serve as a useful clinical marker for the borderline diagnosis, particularly in settings where the base rate of the disorder is high.

We recognize that not all clinicians believe in the existence of defense mechanisms; or even if they do, are not trained to recognize them. Luckily, all three defenses mentioned here are behaviorally oriented, and clinicians can be taught to recognize that acting out is associated with impulsivity, undoing with making amends, and emotional hypochondriasis with insistent and persistent demands that attention be paid to one's inner pain.

DEFENSE MECHANISMS OVER 16 YEARS
OF PROSPECTIVE FOLLOW-UP

Clinicians can also use the defensive functioning of their borderline patients to track their symptomatic progress over time, as we did by studying changes in defensive functioning over a decade and a half (Zanarini, Frankenburg, & Fitzmaurice, 2013). It was found that borderline patients had significantly lower scores than Axis II comparison subjects on one mature defense mechanism (suppression) and significantly higher scores on seven of the other 18 defenses studied. More specifically, borderline patients had significantly higher scores on one neurotic-level defense (undoing), four immature defenses (acting out, emotional hypochondriasis, passive aggression, and projection), and two image-distorting/borderline defenses (projective identification and splitting). In terms of change, borderline patients were found to have had significant improvement on 13 of the 19 defenses studied. More specifically, they had significantly higher scores over time on one mature defense (anticipation) and significantly lower scores on two neurotic defenses (isolation and undoing), all immature defenses, and all image-distorting/borderline defenses except primitive idealization. In addition, four time-varying defense mechanisms were found to predict time-to-recovery (see Table 18.1): humor, acting out, emotional hypochondriasis, and projection.

The results of this study suggest that borderline patients were successfully differentiated from comparison subjects over time by basically the same defenses that differentiated the two study groups at baseline. However, many of the more immature defenses and borderline defenses declined in severity over time—indicating a move toward more adaptive functioning. In addition, four defenses together were significantly related to time-to-recovery. It is not surprising that three of these defenses were immature according to Vaillant's (1986) classification system: acting out, emotional hypochondriasis, and projection. Clearly, continued impulsivity, unremitting complaints of being misunderstood, and chronic distrust and suspiciousness would interfere with both a good social and a good vocational adjustment. However, the fact that humor predicts a faster time to recovery is an unexpected finding. It may be that humor, which requires a well-functioning observing ego, paves the way for a more flexible and mature psychosocial adjustment.

We are well aware that such a focus on assessing change in defense mechanisms as a measure of progress in therapy or life has been replaced in large measure by a focus on emotion dysregulation or maladaptive behaviors associated with such dysregulation. However, this method allows for an emphasis on positive growth or higher levels of adaption to life's challenges and opportunities.

It is important to note that each set of predictors should be viewed as a set. As a good marker for BPD, the clinician should be aware of a high level of impulsivity, which might be indicated by episodes of self-mutilation or suicide attempts; a pattern of insistent and persistent complaints of being misunderstood or uncared for; as well as a pattern of trying to make amends for behavior that causes the borderline patient to feel anxious about abandonment.

In a similar manner, clinicians can use decreasing levels of impulsivity, fewer complaints of being misunderstood, and less frequently seeing a patient's disavowed thoughts and feelings being attributed to others as indicators of recovery from BPD. Increasing levels of humor are also indicative of this positive outcome and may be a sign of finding a more graceful way to deal with all of their inner distress—a more graceful way that takes into account the separateness of the patients and those he or she cares about and needs.

19

Going Forward

We have found that almost all borderline patients achieve at least a two-year symptomatic remission, and that symptomatic recurrences are relatively rare. We have also found that 60% of borderline patients eventually recover, which we have defined as a concurrent remission from BPD and good social and good full-time vocational functioning. In addition, we have found that the suicide rate in this sample is about half that found in older follow-back studies.

We have also found areas with more guarded outcomes, particularly for those with BPD who have not recovered. These areas are poor vocational adjustment and poor physical health.

The 18-year and 20-year follow-up waves have recently been completed. The 22-year wave and the 24-year wave will be completed in a year or so. These new waves of data will allow us to address a number of questions important to those with BPD, their families, and the mental health professionals and primary care physicians treating them. Do recurrences become more common? Do more borderline patients go on to recover?

What percentage lose their recovery? What about additional deaths from suicide or other causes?

Equally important, we have realized that our complex model of borderline psychopathology is a model of the development and maintenance of BPD. What we are lacking is a model of remission and, particularly, recovery. Childhood adversity and adult adversity seem strongly related to the development of certain symptom areas of borderline psychopathology, such as dissociation. However, both remission and recovery seem more related to temperamental factors, premorbid functioning, and innate endowment.

NEW DIRECTIONS

Could it be that other personality features influence a hyperbolic temperament and determine the likelihood of a good or poor outcome? What might these features be? From all of our experience with this study and our patients, it seems that determination and grit might be associated with a good outcome, particularly a recovery from BPD. This is so because other people do not have to motivate or push the person with BPD to try to succeed. They are pushing themselves, and therefore do not waste time and energy resenting others for hoping that they have a fuller life. In a similar fashion, it seems that experiential avoidance might be associated with a poor outcome, particularly in the area of recovery from BPD. This is so because it is difficult to succeed if one is always anxious and if one has learned to avoid anxiety-producing experiences. In many cases, that rules out a social life or a full-time job. Treatment or educational programs to enhance determination and lessen experiential avoidance could be adapted for those with BPD, but clinicians and family members would have to support the introduction of these treatment modules to more standard care. We hope this happens as the long-term course of BPD unfolds.

As a final note, preliminary analyses from our just completed 18-year and 20-year data suggest that very few additional borderline patients attain recovery from BPD. This suggests that there are two stable subgroups or subtypes of borderline patients: those who recover symptomatically and functionally, and those who remit but do not recover. If this observation is true, it might help guide clinical care. It might also help guide the expectations of borderline patients and their family members. As mentioned before, treatment modules for enhancing resilience and reducing experiential avoidance could be developed, but only with support from mental health professionals and family members would these aspects of treatment have any chance of changing the course of BPD. Both require hard work that would stir up the fears of those with BPD, but they could be successful if all of those in the patient's support system could tolerate the distress of the patient, while remaining calm and optimistic. However, it is certainly possible that these modules would not help never-recovered borderline patients become more resilient and less anxiously avoidant. In those cases, the result could be framed as making a good-faith effort to have as rich a life as possible, rather than as a treatment failure.

FINAL THOUGHTS

In that regard, it is simply amazing that 99% of once-borderline inpatients achieve a stable two-year symptomatic remission and that 78% achieve a stable eight-year symptomatic remission. It is also amazing that 60% of these borderline patients achieve a concurrent symptomatic and psychosocial recovery from BPD. These results are unique in psychiatry and would be eye-opening to physicians in other medical specialties, such as endocrinology or gastroenterology, which focus on symptom relief and do not see overcoming psychosocial impairment as part of their clinical responsibilities.

Yet there is much to learn about the course of BPD. And there is much to respect in terms of the persistence evidenced by many borderline patients and the increasingly graceful way that they handle the burdens that their illness imposes upon them.

REFERENCES

Adler, G., & Buie, D. (1979). Aloneness and borderline psychopathology: The possible relevance of child developmental issues. *International Journal of Psychoanalysis, 60*, 83–96.

Akiskal, H. S. (1981). Subaffective disorders: Dysthymic, cyclothymic, and bipolar II disorders in the "borderline" realm. *Psychiatric Clinics of North America, 4*, 25–46.

Akiskal, H. S., Chen, S. E., Davis, G. C., Puzantian, V. R., Kashgarian, M., & Bolinger, J. M. (1985). Borderline: An adjective in search of a noun. *Journal of Clinical Psychiatry, 46*, 41–48.

American Psychiatric Association. (1980). *Diagnostic and Statistical Manual of Mental Disorders* (3rd ed.). Washington, DC: American Psychiatric Association.

American Psychiatric Association. (1987). *Diagnostic and Statistical Manual of Mental Disorders* (3rd ed., revised). Washington, DC: American Psychiatric Association.

American Psychiatric Association. (1994). *Diagnostic and Statistical Manual of Mental Disorders* (4th ed.). Washington, DC: American Psychiatric Association.

American Psychiatric Association. (2013). *Diagnostic and Statistical Manual of Mental Disorders*, (5th ed.). (DSM-5). Arlington, VA: American Psychiatric Publishing.

Antikainen, R., Hintikka, J., Lehtonen, J., Koponen, H., & Arstila, A. (1995). A prospective three-year follow-up study of borderline personality disorder inpatients. *Acta Psychiatrica Scandinavica, 92*, 327–335.

Barasch, A., Frances, A., Hurt, S., Clarkin, J., & Cohen, S. (1985). The stability and distinctness of borderline personality disorder. *American Journal of Psychiatry, 142*, 1484–1486.

Baron, M., Gruen, R., Asnis, L., & Lord, S. (1985). Familial transmission of schizotypal and borderline personality disorders. *American Journal of Psychiatry, 142*, 927–933.

Bateman, A., & Fonagy, P. (1999). Effectiveness of partial hospitalization in the treatment of borderline personality disorder: A randomized controlled trial. *American Journal of Psychiatry, 156*, 1563–1569.

Bender, D. S., Dolan, R. T., Skodol, A. E., Sanislow, C. A., Dyck, I. R., McGlashan, T. H., . . . Gunderson, J. G. (2001). Treatment utilization of patients with personality disorders. *American Journal of Psychiatry, 158*, 295–302.

Bender, D. S., Skodol, A. E., Pagano, M. E., Dyck, I. R., Grilo, C. M., Shea, M. T., . . . Gunderson, J. G. (2006). Prospective assessment of treatment use by patients with personality disorders. *Psychiatric Services, 57,* 254–257.

Bernstein, E. M., & Putnam, F. W. (1986). Development, reliability, and validity of a dissociation scale. *Journal of Nervous and Mental Disease, 174,* 727–735.

Biskin, R. S., Frankenburg, F. R., Fitzmaurice, G. M., & Zanarini, M. C. (2014). Pain in patients with borderline personality disorder. *Personality and Mental Health, 8,* 218–227.

Black, D. W., Zanarini, M. C., Romine, A., Shaw, M., Allen, J., & Schulz, S. C. (2014). Comparison of low and moderate dosages of extended-release quetiapine in borderline personality disorder: A randomized, double-blind, placebo-controlled trial. *American Journal of Psychiatry, 171,* 1174–1182.

Blum, N., St. John, D., Pfohl, B., Stuart, S., McCormick, B., & Allen, J., . . . Black, D. W. (2008). Systems Training for Emotional Predictability and Problem Solving (STEPPS) for outpatients with borderline personality disorder: A randomized controlled trial and 1-year follow-up. *American Journal of Psychiatry, 165,* 468–478.

Bogenschutz, M. P., & Nurnberg, G. H. (2004). Olanzapine versus placebo in the treatment of borderline personality disorder. *Journal of Clinical Psychiatry, 65,* 104–109.

Bond, M. (1990). Are "borderline defenses" specific for borderline personality disorders? *Journal of Personality Disorders, 4,* 251–256.

Bond, M. (1991). *Manual for the Defense Style Questionnaire.* Montreal: McGill University.

Bond, M. (1992). *An Empirical Study of Defensive Styles: The Defense Style Questionnaire.* In G. E. Vaillant (Ed.), *Ego Mechanisms of Defense* (pp. 127–158). Washington, DC: American Psychiatric Press.

Bond, M., Paris, J., & Zweig-Frank, H. (1994). Defense styles and borderline personality disorder. *Journal of Personality Disorders, 8,* 28–31.

Bradley, S. J. (1979). The relationship of early maternal separation to borderline personality in children and adolescents: A pilot study. *American Journal of Psychiatry, 136,* 424–426.

Brodsky, B. S., Cloitre, M., & Dulit, R. A. (1995). Relationship of dissociation to self-mutilation and childhood abuse in borderline personality disorder. *American Journal of Psychiatry, 152,* 1788–1792.

Burnham, D. (1966). The special problem patient: Victim or agent of splitting? *Psychiatry, 29,*105–122.

Carpenter, J. S., & Andrykowski, M. A. (1998). Psychometric evaluation of the Pittsburgh Sleep Quality Index. *Journal of Psychosomatic Research, 45,* 5–13.

Carpenter, W. T., & Gunderson, J. G. (1977). Five year follow-up comparison of borderline and schizophrenic patients. *Comprehensive Psychiatry, 18,* 567–571.

Clarkin, J. F., Hull, J. W., Cantor, J., & Sanderson, C. (1993). Borderline personality disorder and personality traits: A comparison of SCID-II BPD and NEO-PI. *Psychological Assessment, 5,* 472–476.

Clarkin, J. F., Levy, K. N., Lenzenweger, M. F., & Kernberg, O. F. (2007). Evaluating three treatments for borderline personality: A multiwave study. *American Journal of Psychiatry, 164,* 922–928.

Coccaro, E. F., Siever, L. J., Klar, H. M., Maurer, G., Cochrane, K., Cooper, T. B., . . . Davis, K. L. (1989). Serotonergic studies in affective and personality disorders: Correlates with suicidal and impulsive aggressive behavior. *Archives of General Psychiatry, 46,* 587–599.

Coryell, W., Endicott, J., Maser, J. D., Mueller, T., Lavori, P., & Keller, M. (1995). The likelihood of recurrence in bipolar affective disorder; the importance of episode recency. *Journal of Affective Disorders, 14,* 201–206.

Costa, P. T., & McCrae, R. R. (1992). *Revised NEO Personality Inventory and NEO Five-Factor Inventory Professional Manual.* Odessa, FL: Psychological Assessment Resources.

Cowdry, R., & Gardner, D. L. (1988). Pharmacotherapy of borderline personality disorder-alprazolam, carbamazepine, trifluoperazine, and tranylcypromine. *Archives of General Psychiatry, 45,* 111–119.

Deutsch, H. (1942). Some forms of emotional disturbance and their relationship to schizophrenia. *Psychoanalytic Quarterly, 11,* 301–321.

Endicott, J., Spitzer, R. L., Fleiss, J. L., & Cohen, J. (1976). The Global Assessment Scale: A procedure for measuring overall severity of psychiatric disturbance. *Archives of General Psychiatry, 33,* 766–771.

Frank, H., & Hoffman, N. (1986). Borderline empathy: An empirical investigation. *Comprehensive Psychiatry, 27,* 387–395.

Frank, H., & Paris, J. (1981). Recollections of family experience in borderline patients. *Archives of General Psychiatry, 38,* 1031–1034.

Frankenburg, F. R., Fitzmaurice, G. M., & Zanarini, M. C. (2014). The use of prescription opioid medication by patients with borderline personality disorder and Axis II comparison subjects: A 10-year follow-up study. *Journal of Clinical Psychiatry, 75,* 357–361.

Frankenburg, F. R., & Zanarini, M. C. (2002). Divalproex sodium treatment of women with borderline personality disorder and bipolar II disorder: A double-blind placebo-controlled pilot study. *Journal of Clinical Psychiatry, 63,* 442–446.

Frankenburg, F. R., & Zanarini, M. C. (2004a). *Medical History and Services Utilization Interview (MHSUI).* Belmont, MA: McLean Hospital.

Frankenburg, F. R., & Zanarini, M. C. (2004b). The association between borderline personality disorder and chronic medical illnesses, poor health-related life style choices, and costly forms of health care utilization. *Journal of Clinical Psychiatry, 65,* 1660–1665.

Frankenburg, F. R., & Zanarini, M. C. (2006). Obesity and obesity-related illnesses in borderline patients. *Journal of Personality Disorders, 20,* 71–80.

Frankenburg, F. R., & Zanarini, M. C. (2011). Relationship between cumulative BMI and symptomatic, psychosocial, and medical outcomes in patients with borderline personality disorder. *Journal of Personality Disorders, 25,* 421–431.

Freud, A. (1937). *The Ego and the Mechanisms of Defense.* London: Hogarth Press.

Frosch, J. (1960). The psychotic character. *Journal of the American Psychoanalytic Association, 8,* 544–551.

Giesen-Bloo, J., van Dyck, R., Spinhoven, P., van Tilburg, W., Dirksen, C., van Asselt, T., . . . Arntz, A. (2006). Outpatient psychotherapy for borderline personality disorder: Randomized trial of schema-focused therapy vs. transference-focused psychotherapy. *Archives of General Psychiatry, 63,* 649–658.

Goldberg, R. L., Mann, L. S., Wise, T. N., & Segall, E. A. (1985). Parental qualities as perceived by borderline personality disorders. *Hillside Journal of Clinical Psychiatry, 7,* 134–140.

Grinker, R. R., Werble, B., & Drye, R. C. (1968). *The Borderline Syndrome: A Behavioral Study of Ego-functions.* New York: Basic Books.

Gunderson, J. G. (1984). *Borderline Personality Disorder.* Washington, DC: American Psychiatric Press

Gunderson, J. G., Carpenter, W. T., & Strauss, J. S. (1975). Borderline and schizophrenic patients: A comparative study. *American Journal of Psychiatry, 132,* 1257–1264.

Gunderson, J., Kerr, J., & Englund, D. (1980). The families of borderlines: A comparative study. *Archives of General Psychiatry, 37,* 27–33.

Gunderson, J. G., & Kolb, J. E. (1978). Discriminating features of borderline patients. *American Journal Psychiatry, 135,* 792–796.

Gunderson, J. G., Kolb, J. E., & Austin, V. (1981). The diagnostic interview for borderline patients. *American Journal of Psychiatry, 138,* 896–903.

Gunderson, J. G., & Links, P. S. (2008). *Borderline Personality Disorder: A Clinical Guide,* (2nd ed.). Washington, DC: American Psychiatric Publishing.

Gunderson, J. G., & Singer, M. T. (1975). Defining borderline patients: An overview. *American Journal of Psychiatry, 132,* 1–10.

Gunderson, J. G., Stout, R. L., McGlashan, T. H., Shea, M. T., Morey, L. C., Grilo, C. M., . . . Skodol, A. E. (2011). Ten-year course of borderline personality disorder: Psychopathology and function from the Collaborative Longitudinal Personality Disorders Study. *Archives of General Psychiatry, 68,* 827–837.

Gunderson, J. G., Zanarini, M. C., Choi-Kain, L. W., Mitchell, K. S., Jang, K. L., & Hudson, J. I. (2011). Family study of borderline personality disorder and its sectors of psychopathology. *Archives of General Psychiatry, 68,* 753–762.

Ha, C., Balderas, J. C., Zanarini, M. C., Oldham, J., & Sharp, C. (2014). Psychiatric comorbidity in hospitalized adolescents with borderline personality disorder. *Journal of Clinical Psychiatry, 75,* 457–464.

Herman, J. L. (1986). Histories of violence in an outpatient population: An exploratory study. *American Journal of Orthopsychiatry, 56,* 137–141.

Herman, J. L., & Van Der Kolk, B. A. (1987). Traumatic antecedents of borderline personality disorder. In B. A. van der Kolk (Ed.), *Psychological Trauma* (pp. 111–126). Washington, DC: American Psychiatric Press.

Herman, J. L., Perry, J. C., & van der Kolk, B. A. (1989). Childhood trauma in borderline personality disorder. *American Journal of Psychiatry, 146,* 490–495.

Hoch, P. H., & Polatin, P. (1949). Pseudoneurotic forms of schizophrenia. *Psychiatric Quarterly, 23,* 248–276.

Hoffman, P. D., Fruzzetti, A. E., & Buteau, E. (2007). Understanding and engaging families: An education, skills and support program for relatives impacted by Borderline Personality Disorder. *Journal of Mental Health, 16,* 69–82.

Hollander, E., Allen, A., Lopez, R. P., Bienstock, C. A., Grossman, R., Siever, L. J., . . . Stein, D. J. (2001). A preliminary double-blind, placebo-controlled trial of divalproex sodium in borderline personality disorder. *Journal of Clinical Psychiatry, 62,* 199–203.

Hollander, E., Stein, D. J., Decaria, C. M., Cohen, L., Saoud, J. B., Skodol, A. E., . . . Oldham, J. M. (1994). Serotonergic sensitivity in borderline personality disorder: Preliminary findings. *American Journal of Psychiatry, 151,* 277–280.

Hollander, E., Swann, A. C., Coccaro, E. F., Jiang, P., & Smith, T. B. (2005). Impact of trait impulsivity and state aggression on divalproex versus placebo response in borderline personality disorder. *American Journal of Psychiatry, 162,* 621–624.

Hollingshead, A. B. (1957). *Two Factor Index of Social Position.* New Haven, CT: Yale University.

Hooley, J. M., & Hoffman, P. D. (1999). Expressed emotion and clinical outcome in borderline personality disorder. *American Journal of Psychiatry, 156,* 1557–1562.

Hörz, S., Zanarini, M. C., Frankenburg, F. R., Reich, D. B., & Fitzmaurice, G. M. (2010). Ten-year use of mental health services by patients with borderline personality disorder and with other axis II disorders. *Psychiatric Services, 61,* 612–616.

Jang, K. L., Paris, J., Zweig-Frank, H., & Livesley, W. J. (1998). Twin study of dissociative experience. *Journal of Nervous and Mental Disease, 186,* 345–351.

Jang, K. L., Livesley, W. J., & Vernon, P. A. (1996). Heritability of the Big Five personality dimensions and their facets: A twin study. *Journal of Personality, 64,* 577–591.

Jang, K. L., McCrae, R. R., Angleitner, A., Reimann, R., & Livesley, W. J. (1998). Heritability of facet-level traits in a cross-cultural twin sample: Support for a hierarchical model. *Journal of Personality and Social Psychology, 74,* 1556–1565.

Karan, E., Niesten, I. J. M., Frankenburg, F. R., Fitzmaurice, G. M., & Zanarini, M. C. (2014). The 16-year course of shame and its risk factors in patients with borderline personality disorder. *Personality and Mental Health, 8,* 169–177.

Karan, E., Niesten, I. J. M., Frankenburg, F. R., Fitzmaurice, G. M., & Zanarini, M. C. (2016). Prevalence and course of sexual relationship difficulties in recovered and non-recovered patients with borderline personality disorder over 16 years of prospective follow-up. *Personality and Mental Health, 10,* 232–243.

Kendler, K. S., Myers, J., & Reichborn-Kjennerud, T. (2011). Borderline personality disorder traits and their relationship with dimensions of normative personality: A web-based cohort and twin study. *Acta Psychiatrica Scandinavica, 123,* 349–359.

Kernberg, O. F. (1967). Borderline personality organization. *Journal of American Psychoanalytic Association, 15,* 641–685.

Keuroghlian, A. S., Frankenburg, F. R., & Zanarini, M. C. (2013). The relationship of chronic medical illnesses, poor health-related lifestyle choices, and health care utilization to recovery status in borderline patients over a decade of prospective follow-up. *Journal of Psychiatric Research, 47,* 1499–1506.

Knight, R. P. (1953). Borderline states. *Bulletin Menninger Clinic, 17,* 1–12.

Kochanek, K. D., Murphy, S. L., Xu, J. Q., & Tejada-Vera, B. (2016). *Deaths: Final Data for 2014.* Hyattsville, MD: National Center for Health Statistics.

Lezenweger, M. F., Lane, M. C., Loranger, A. W., & Kessler, R. C. (2007). DSM-IV personality disorders in the National Comorbidity Survey replication. *Biological Psychiatry, 62,* 553–564.

Linehan, M. M. (1993). *Cognitive-Behavioral Treatment of Borderline Personality Disorder.* New York: Guilford Press.

Linehan, M. M., Armstrong, H. E., Suarez, A., Allmon, D., & Heard, H. L. (1991). Cognitive-behavioral treatment of chronically parasuicidal borderline patients. *Archives of General Psychiatry, 48,* 1060–1064.

Linehan, M. M., Heard, H. L., & Armstrong, H. F. (1993). Naturalistic follow-up of a behavioral treatment for chronically parasuicidal borderline patients. *Archives of General Psychiatry, 50,* 971–974.

Linehan, M. M., Schmidt, H., Dimeff, L. A., Craft, J. C., Kanter, J., & Comtois, K. A. (1999). Dialectical behavioral therapy for patients with borderline personality disorder and drug-dependence. *American Journal on Addictions, 8,* 279–292.

Links, P. S., Heslegrave, R. J., & Van Reekum, R. (1998). Prospective follow-up study of borderline personality disorder: Prognosis, prediction of outcome, and axis II co-morbidity. *Canadian Journal of Psychiatry, 42,* 265–270.

Links, P. S., Heslegrave, R., & van Reekum, R. (1999). Impulsivity: Core aspect of borderline personality disorder. *Journal of Personality Disorders, 13,* 1–9.

Links, P. S., Heslegrave, R. J., Mitton, J. E., Van Reekum, R., & Patrick, J. (1995). Borderline psychopathology and recurrences of clinical disorders. *Journal of Nervous and Mental Disease, 183,* 582–586.

Links, P. S., Mitton, J. E., & Steiner, M. (1990). Predicting outcome for borderline personality disorder. *Comprehensive Psychiatry, 31,* 490–498.

Links, P. S., Steiner, M., & Huxley, G. (1988). The occurrence of borderline personality disorder in the families of borderline patients. *Journal of Personality Disorders, 2,* 14–20.

Links, P. S., Steiner, M., Offord, D. R., & Eppel, A. (1988). Characteristics of borderline personality disorder: A Canadian study. *Canadian Journal of Psychiatry, 33,* 336–340.

Loew, T. H., Nickel, M. K., Muehlbacher, M., Kaplan, P., Nickel, C., Kettler, C., . . . Egger, C. (2006). Topiramate treatment for women with borderline personality disorder: A double-blind, placebo study. *Journal of Clinical Psycho-pharmacology, 26,* 61–66.

Loranger, A. W., Oldham, J. M., & Tulis, E. H. (1982). Familial transmission of DSM-III borderline personality disorder. *Archives of General Psychiatry, 39,* 795–799.

Luborsky, L. (1962). Clinician's judgements of mental health: A proposed scale. *Archives General Psychiatry, 7,* 407–417.

Mahler, M. (1971). A study of the separation-individuation process and its possible application to borderline phenomena in the psychoanalytic situation. *Psychoanalytic Study of the Child, 26,* 403–424.

Main, T. (1957). The ailment. *British Journal of Medical Psychology, 30,* 129–145.

Maltsberger, J., & Buie, D. (1974). Countertransference hatred in the treatment of suicidal patients. *Archives General Psychiatry, 30,* 625–633.

Marino, M. F., & Zanarini, M. C. (2001). Subtypes of eating disorder NOS comorbid with borderline personality disorder. *International Journal of Eating Disorders, 29,* 349–353

Masterson, J. (1972). *Treatment of the Borderline Adolescent: A Developmental Approach.* New York: Wiley.

McGlashan, T. H. (1985). The prediction of outcome in borderline personality disorder: Part V of the Chestnut Lodge follow-up study. In: McGlashan, T. H. (Ed.), *The Borderline: Current Empirical Research* (pp. 63–098). Washington, DC: American Psychiatric Press.

McGlashan, T. H. (1986). The Chestnut Lodge follow-up study: III. Long-term outcome of borderline personalities. *Archives of General Psychiatry, 43,* 20–30.

McGlashan, T. H., Grilo, C. M., Sanislow, C. A., Ralevski, E., Morey, L. C., Gunderson, J. G., . . . Pagano, M. (2005). Two-year prevalence and stability of individual criteria for schizotypal, borderline, avoidant, and obsessive-compulsive personality disorders. *American Journal of Psychiatry, 162,* 883–889.

McGowan, A., King, H., Frankenburg, F. R., Fitzmaurice, G. M., & Zanarini, M. C. (2012). The course of adult experiences of abuse in patients with borderline personality disorder and axis II comparison subjects: A 10-year follow-up study. *Journal of Personality Disorders, 26,* 192–202.

McMain, S. F., Links, P. S., Gnam, W. H., Guimond, T., Cardish, R. J., Korman, L., & Streiner, D. L. (2009). A randomized trial of dialectical behavior therapy versus general psychiatric management for borderline personality disorder. *American Journal of Psychiatry, 166,* 1365–1374.

Mehlum, L., Friis, S., Irion, T., Johns, S., Karterud, S., Vaglum, P., & Vaglum, S. (1991). Personality disorders 2–5 years after treatment: A prospective follow-up study. *Acta Psychiatrica Scandinavica, 84,* 72–77.

Modestin, J., & Villiger, C. (1989). Follow-up study on borderline versus nonborderline disorders. *Comprehensive Psychiatry, 30,* 236–244.

Morey, L. C., & Zanarini, M. C. (2000). Borderline personality traits and disorder. *Journal of Abnormal Psychology, 109,* 733–737.

Morin, C. M., Vallières, A., & Ivers, H. (2007). Dysfunctional Beliefs and Attitudes About Sleep (DBAS): Validation of a brief version (DBAS-16). *Sleep, 30,* 1547–1554.

Mueller, T. I., Leon, A. A. C., Keller, M. B., Solomon, D. A., Endicott, J., Coryell, W., Warshaw, M., & Maser, J. D. (1999). Recurrence after recovery from major depressive disorder during 15 years of observational follow-up. *American Journal of Psychiatry, 156,* 1000–1006.

Nace, E. P., Saxon, J. J., & Shore, N. (1986). Borderline personality disorder and alcoholism treatment: A one-year follow-up study. *Journal of Studies on Alcohol, 47,* 196–200.

Najavits, L. M., & Gunderson, J. G. (1995). Better than expected: Improvements in borderline personality disorder in a 3-year prospective outcome study. *Comprehensive Psychiatry, 36,* 296–302.

Nickel, M. K., Nickel, C., Mitterlehner, F. O., Tritt, K., Lahmann, C., Leiberich, P. K., . . . Loew, T. H. (2004). Topiramate treatment of aggression in female borderline personality disorder patients: A double blind placebo-controlled study. *Journal of Clinical Psychiatry, 65,* 1515–1519.

Nickel, M. K., Nickel, C., Kaplan, P., Lahmann, C., Muhlbacher, M., Tritt, K., . . . Loew, T. H. (2005). Treatment of aggression with topiramate in male borderline patients: A double-blind, placebo-controlled study. *Biological Psychiatry, 57,* 495–499.

Niesten, I. J. M., Karan, E., Frankenburg, F. R., Fitzmaurice, G. M., & Zanarini, M. C. (2014). Prevalence and risk factors for irritable bowel syndrome in recovered and non-recovered borderline patients over ten years of prospective follow-up. *Personality and Mental Health*, *8*, 14–23.

Ogata, S. N., Silk, K. R., Goodrich, S., Lohr, N. E., Westen, D., & Hill, E. M. (1990). Childhood sexual and physical abuse in adult patients with borderline personality disorder. *American Journal of Psychiatry*, *147*, 1008–1013.

Paris, J., Brown, R., & Nowlis, D. (1987). Long-term follow-up of borderline patients in a general hospital. *Comprehensive Psychiatry*, *28*, 530–535.

Paris, J., & Frank, H. (1989). Perceptions of parental bonding in borderline patients. *American Journal of Psychiatry*, *146*, 1498–1499.

Paris, J., Nowlis, D., & Brown, R. (1988). Developmental factors in the outcome of borderline personality disorder. *Comprehensive Psychiatry*, *29*, 147–150.

Paris, J., & Zweig-Frank, H. (2001). A 27-year follow-up of patients with borderline personality disorder. *Comprehensive Psychiatry*, *42*, 482–487.

Paris, J., Zweig-Frank, H., & Guzder, J. (1994a). Psychological risk factors for borderline personality disorder in female patients. *Comprehensive Psychiatry*, *35*, 301–305.

Paris, J., Zweig-Frank, H., & Guzder, J. (1994b). Risk factors for borderline personality in male outpatients. *Journal of Nervous and Mental Disease*, *182*, 375–380.

Perry, J., & Cooper, S. (1985). Psychodynamic symptoms and outcome in borderline and antisocial personality disorders and bipolar II affective disorder. In *The Borderline: Current Empirical Research* (pp. 21–41). Washington, DC: American Psychiatric Press.

Perry, J. C., & Cooper, S. H. (1986). A preliminary report on defenses and conflicts associated with borderline personality disorder. *Journal of American Psychoanalysis Association*, *34*, 863–893.

Plakun, E. M. (1991). Prediction of outcome in borderline personality disorder. *Journal of Personality Disorders*, *5*, 93–101.

Plakun, E. M., Burkhardt, P. E., & Muller, J. P. (1985). 14-year follow-up of borderline and schizotypal personality disorders. *Comprehensive Psychiatry*, *26*, 448–455.

Plante, D. T., Frankenburg, F. R., Fitzmaurice, G. M., & Zanarini, M. C. (2013a). Relationship between sleep disturbance and recovery in patients with borderline personality disorder. *Journal of Psychosomatic Research*, *74*, 278–282.

Plante, D. T., Frankenburg, F. R., Fitzmaurice, G. M., & Zanarini, M. C. (2013b). Relationship between maladaptive cognitions about sleep and recovery in patients with borderline personality disorder. *Psychiatry Research*, *30*, 975–979.

Plante, D. T., Zanarini, M. C., Frankenburg, F. R., & Fitzmaurice, G. M. (2009). Sedative-hypnotic use in patients with borderline personality disorder and axis II comparison subjects. *Journal of Personality Disorders*, *23*, 563–571.

Pope, H. G., Jonas, J. M., Hudson, J. I., Cohen, B. M., & Gunderson, J. G. (1983). The validity of DSM-III borderline personality disorder: A phenomenologic, family history, treatment response, and long-term follow- up study. *Archives General Psychiatry*, *40*, 23–30.

Pope, H. G., Jonas, J. M., Hudson, J. I., Cohen, B. M., & Tohen, M. (1985). An empirical study of psychosis in borderline personality disorder. *American Journal Psychiatry*, *142*, 1285–1290.

Reed, L. I., & Zanarini, M. C. (2011). Positive affective and cognitive states in borderline personality disorder. *Journal of Personality Disorders*, *25*, 851–862.

Reich, D. B., & Zanarini, M. C. (2001). Developmental aspects of borderline personality disorder. *Harvard Review of Psychiatry*, *9*, 294–301.

Reich, D. B., & Zanarini, M. C. (2008). Sexual orientation and relationship choice in borderline personality disorder over ten years of prospective follow-up. *Journal of Personality Disorders*, *22*, 564–572.

Reichborn-Kjennerud, T., Ystrom, E., Neale, M. C., Aggen, S. H., Mazzeo, S. E., Knudsen, G. P., . . . Kendler, K. S. (2013). Structure of genetic and environmental risk factors for symptoms of DSM-IV borderline personality disorder. *Journal of American Medical Association Psychiatry*, *70*, 1206–1214.

Rinne, T., van den Brink, W., Wouters, L., & van Dyck, R. (2002). SSRI treatment of borderline personality disorder: A randomized placebo-controlled clinical trial for female patients with borderline personality disorder. *American Journal of Psychiatry*, *159*, 2048–2054.

Robins, L. N. (1966). *Deviant Children Grown Up: A Sociological and Psychiatric Study of Sociopathic Personality*. Baltimore, MD: Williams & Wilkins.

Robins, E., & Guze, S. B. (1970). Establishment of diagnostic validity in psychiatric illness: Its application to schizophrenia. *American Journal of Psychiatry*, *126*, 983–987.

Salzman, J. P., Salzman, C., Wolfson, A. N., Albanese, M., Looper, J., Ostacher, M., . . . Miyawaki, E. (1993). Association between borderline personality structure and history of childhood abuse in adult volunteers. *Comprehensive Psychiatry*, *34*, 254–257.

Salzman, C., Wolfson, A. N., Schatzberg, A., Looper, J., Henke, R., Albanese, M., . . . Miyawki, E. (1995). Effect of fluoxetine on anger in symptomatic volunteers with borderline personality disorder. *Journal of Clinical Psychopharmacology*, *15*, 23–29.

Sandell, R., Alfredsson, E., Berg, M., Crafoord, K., Lagerlof, A., Arkel, I., . . . Rugolska, A. (1993). Clinical significance of outcome in long-term follow-up of borderline patients at a day hospital. *Acta Psychiatrica Scandinavica*, *87*, 405–413.

Senol, S., Dereboy, C., & Yuksel, N. (1997). Borderline disorder in Turkey: A 2- to 4-year follow-up. *Social Psychiatry and Psychiatric Epidemiology*, *32*, 109–112.

Schmideberg, M. (1947). The treatment of psychopaths and borderline patients. *American Journal of Psychotherapy*, *1*, 45–70.

Schulz, S. C., Camlin, K. L., Berry, S., & Friedman, L. (1999). Risperidone for borderline personality disorder: A double-blind study. In *Proceedings of the 39th Annual Meeting of the American College of Neuropsychopharmacology*. Nashville, TN: ACNP.

Schulz, S. C., Zanarini, M. C., Bateman, A., Bohus, M., Detke, H. C., Trzaskoma, Q., . . . Corya, S. (2008). Olanzapine for the treatment of borderline personality disorder: A variable-dose, 12-week, randomized, double-blind, placebo-controlled study. *British Journal of Psychiatry*, *193*, 485–492.

Shea, M. T., Edelen, M. O., Pinto, A., Yen, S., Gunderson, J. G., Skodol, A. E., . . . Morey, L. C. (2009). Improvement in borderline personality disorder in relationship to age. *Acta Psychiatrica Scandinavica, 119*, 143–148.

Shea, M. T., Stout, R. L., Gunderson, J. G., Morey, L. C., Grilo, C. M., McGlashan, T. H., & Keller, M. B. (2002). Short-term diagnostic stability of schizotypal, borderline, avoidant, and obsessive-compulsive personality disorders. *American Journal of Psychiatry, 159*, 2036–2041.

Shearer, S. L. (1994). Dissociative phenomena in women with borderline personality disorder. *American Journal Psychiatry, 151*, 1324–1328.

Shearer, S. L., Peters, C. P., Quaytman, M. S., & Ogden, R. L. (1990). Frequency and correlates of childhood sexual and physical abuse histories in adult female borderline inpatients. *American Journal of Psychiatry, 147*, 214–216.

Shrout, P. E., Link, B. G., Dohrenwend, B. P., Skodol, A. E., Stueve, A., & Mirotznik, J. (1989). Characterizing life events as risk factors for depression: The role of fateful loss events. *Journal of Abnormal Psychology, 98*, 460–467.

Siever, L. J., & Davis, K. L. (1991). A psychobiological perspective on the personality disorders. *American Journal of Psychiatry, 148*, 1647–1658.

Silverman, M. H., Frankenburg, F. R., Reich, D. B., Fitzmaurice, G. M., & Zanarini, M. C. (2012). The course of anxiety disorders other than PTSD in patients with borderline personality disorder and axis II comparison subjects: A 10-year follow-up study. *Journal Personality Disorders, 26*, 804–814.

Silverman, J. M., Pinkham, L., Horvath, T. B., Coccaro, E. F., Klar, H., Schear, S., . . . Siever, L. J. (1991). Affective and impulsive personality disorder traits in the relatives of patients with borderline personality disorder. *American Journal of Psychiatry, 148*, 1378–1385.

Skodol, A. E., Gunderson, J. G., McGlashan, T. H., Dyck, I. R., Stout, R. L., Bender, D. S., . . . Oldham, J. M. (2002). Functional impairment in schizotypal, borderline, avoidant, and obsessive-compulsive personality disorders. *American Journal of Psychiatry, 159*, 276–283.

Skodol, A. E., Pagano, M. E., Bender, D. S., Shea, M. T., Gunderson, J. G., Yen, S., . . . McGlashan, T. H. (2005). Stability of functional impairment in patients with schizotypal, borderline, avoidant, or obsessive-compulsive personality disorder over two years. *Psychological Medicine, 35*, 443–451.

Solomon, D. A., Keller, M. B., Leon, A. C., Mueller, T. I., Shea, M. T., Warshaw, M., . . . Endicott, J. (1997). Recovery from major depression: A 10-year prospective follow-up across multiple episodes. *Archives of General Psychiatry, 54*, 989–991.

Soler, J., Pascual, J. C., Campins, J., Barrachina, J., Puigdemont, D., Alvarez, E., . . . Perez, V. (2005). Double-blind, placebo-controlled study of dialectical behavior therapy plus olanzapine for borderline personality disorder. *American Journal of Psychiatry, 162*, 1221–1224.

Soloff, P. H., Cornelius, J., George, A., Nathan, S., Perel, J. M., & Ulrich, R. F. (1993). Efficacy of phenelzine and haloperidol in borderline personality disorder. *Archives of General Psychiatry, 50*, 377–385.

Soloff, P. H., George, A., Nathan, R. S., Schulz, P. M., Cornelius, J. R., Herring, J., & Perel, J. M. (1989). Amitriptyline versus haloperidol in borderlines: Final outcomes and predictors of response. *Journal of Clinical Psychopharmacology, 9*, 238–246.

Soloff, P. H., & Millward, J. W. (1983). Developmental histories of borderline patients. *Comprehensive Psychiatry, 24*, 574–588.

Spitzer, R. L., Endicott, J., & Gibbon, M. (1979). Crossing the border into borderline personality and borderline schizophrenia. *Archives of General Psychiatry, 36*, 17–24.

Spitzer, R. L., Williams, J. B., Gibbon, M., & First, M. B. (1992). Structured Clinical Interview for DSM-III-R (SCID). I: History, rationale, and description. *Archives of General Psychiatry, 49*, 624–629.

Stern, A. (1938). Psychoanalytic investigation of and therapy in the borderline group of neuroses. *Psychoanalytic Quarterly, 7*, 467–489.

Stevenson, J., & Meares, R. (1992). An outcome study of psychotherapy for patients with borderline personality disorder. *American Journal of Psychiatry, 149*, 358–362.

Stone, M. H. (1980). *The Borderline Syndromes: Constitution, Personality, and Adaptation.* New York: McGraw-Hill.

Stone, M. H. (1990). *The Fate of Borderline Patients.* New York: Guilford Press.

Swartz, M., Blazer, D., George, L., & Winfield, I. (1990). Estimating the prevalence of borderline personality disorder in the community. *Journal of Personality Disorders, 4*, 257–272.

Tohen, M., Hennen, J., Zarate, C. M., Baldessarini, R. J., Strakowski, S. M., Stoll, A. L., . . . Cohen, B. M. (2000). Two-year syndromal and functional recovery in 219 cases of first-episode major affective disorder with psychotic features. *American Journal of Psychiatry, 157*, 220–228.

Torgersen, S., Lygren, S., Oien, P. A., Skre, I., Onstad, S., Evvardsen, J., . . . Kringlen, E. (2000). A twin study of personality disorders. *Comprehensive Psychiatry, 41*, 416–425.

Torgerson, S., Myers, J., Reichborn-Kjennerud, T., Røysamb, E., Kubarych, T. S., & Kendler, K. S. (2012). The heritability of cluster B personality disorders assessed both by personal interview and questionnaire. *Journal of Personality Disorders, 26*, 848–866.

Tritt, K., Nickel, C., Lahmann, C., Leiberich, P. K., Rother, W. K., Loew, T. H., . . . Nickel, M. K. (2005). Lamotrigine treatment of aggression in female borderline-patients: A randomized, double-blind, placebo-controlled study. *Journal of Psychopharmacology, 19*, 287–291.

Trull, T. J., Jahng, S., Tomko, R. L., Wood, P. K., & Sher, K. J. (2010). Revised NESARC personality disorder diagnoses: Gender, prevalence, and comorbidity with substance dependence disorders. *Journal of Personality Disorders, 24*, 412–426.

Trull, T. J., Widiger, T. A., Lynam, D. R., & Costa, P. T. (2003). Borderline personality disorder from the perspective of general personality functioning. *Journal of Abnormal Psychology, 112*, 193–202.

Tucker, L., Bauer, S. F., Wagner, S., Harlam, D., & Sher, I. (1987). Long-term hospital treatment of borderline patients: A descriptive outcome study. *American Journal of Psychiatry, 144*, 1443–1448.

Vaillant, G. E. (1977). *Adaption to Life.* Cambridge, MA: Harvard University Press.

Vaillant, G. E., Bond, M., & Vaillant, C. O. (1986). An empirically validated hierarchy of defense mechanisms. *Archives of General Psychiatry, 43,* 786–794.

Walsh, F. (1977). The family of the borderline patient. In R. R. Grinker & B. Werble (Eds.), *The Borderline Patient* (pp. 149–177). New York: Jason Aronson.

Wedig, M. M., Frankenburg, F. R., Reich, B. D., Fitzmaurice, G. M., & Zanarini, M. C. (2013). Predictors of suicide threats in patients with borderline personality disorder over 16 years of prospective follow-up. *Psychiatry Research, 208,* 252–256.

Wedig, M. M., Silverman, M. H., Frankenburg, F. R., Reich, D. B., Fitzmaurice, G. M., & Zanarini, M. C. (2012). Predictors of suicide attempts in patients with borderline personality disorder over 16 years of prospective follow-up. *Psychological Medicine, 42,* 2395–2404.

Werble, B. (1970). Second follow-up study of borderline patients. *Archives General Psychiatry, 23,* 1–7.

Westen, D., Ludolph, P., Misle, B., Ruffins, S., & Block, J. (1990). Physical and sexual abuse in adolescent girls with borderline personality disorder. *American Journal of Orthopsychiatry, 60,* 55–66.

Widiger, T. A., & Frances, A. J. (1989). Epidemiology, diagnosis, and comorbidity of borderline personality disorder. In A. Tasman, R. E. Hales, & A. Frances (Eds.), *Review of Psychiatry* (Vol. 8, pp. 8–24). Washington, DC: American Psychiatric Press.

Wilberg, T., Urnes, O., Friis, S., Pederson, G., & Karterud, S. (1999). Borderline and avoidant personality disorders and the five-factor model of personality: A comparison between DSM-IV diagnoses and NEO-PI-R. *Journal of Personality Disorders, 13,* 226–240.

Zachary, R. A. (1994). *Shipley Institute of Living Scale: Revised Manual.* Los Angeles, CA: Western Psychological Services.

Zanarini, M. C., Barison, L. K., Frankenburg, F. R., Reich, D. B., & Hudson, J. I. (2009). Family history study of the familial coaggregation of borderline personality disorder with axis I and non-dramatic cluster axis II disorders. *Journal Personality Disorders, 23,* 357–369.

Zanarini, M. C., Conkey, L. C., Temes, C. M., & Fitzmaurice, G. M. (2017 Jul 11 Epub ahead of print). Randomized, controlled trial of web-based psychoeducation for women with borderline personality disorder. *Journal of Clinical Psychiatry.*

Zanarini, M. C., & Frankenburg, F. R. (1994). Emotional hypochondriasis, hyperbole, and the borderline patient. *Journal of Psychotherapy Practice and Research, 3,* 25–36.

Zanarini, M. C., & Frankenburg, F. R. (1997). Pathways to the development of borderline personality disorder. *Journal of Personality Disorders, 11,* 93–104.

Zanarini, M. C., & Frankenburg, F. R. (2001a). Attainment and maintenance of reliability of axis I and II disorders over the course of a longitudinal study. *Comprehensive Psychiatry, 42,* 369–374.

Zanarini, M. C., & Frankenburg, F. R. (2001b). Olanzapine treatment of female borderline personality disorder patients: A double-blind, placebo-controlled pilot study. *Journal of Clinical Psychiatry, 62,* 849–854.

Zanarini, M. C., & Frankenburg, F. R. (2003). Omega-3 fatty acid treatment of women with borderline personality disorder: A double-blind, placebo-controlled pilot study. *American Journal of Psychiatry, 160,* 167–169.

Zanarini, M. C., Frankenburg, F. R., Chauncey, D. L., & Gunderson, J. G. (1987). The Diagnostic Interview for Personality Disorders: Interrater and test-retest reliability. *Comprehensive Psychiatry, 28,* 467–480.

Zanarini, M. C., Frankenburg, F. R., DeLuca, C. J., Hennen, J., Khera, G. S., & Gunderson, J. G. (1998). The pain of being borderline: Dysphoric states specific to borderline personality disorder. *Harvard Review of Psychiatry, 6,* 201–207.

Zanarini, M. C., Frankenburg, F. R., Dubo, E. D., Sickel, A. E., Trikha, A., Levin, A., & Reynolds, V. (1998a). The axis II comorbidity of borderline personality disorder. *Comprehensive Psychiatry, 39,* 296–302.

Zanarini, M. C., Frankenburg, F. R., Dubo, E. D., Sickel, A. E., Trikha, A., Levin, A., & Reynolds, V. (1998b). The axis I comorbidity of borderline personality disorder. *American Journal of Psychiatry, 155,* 1733–1739.

Zanarini, M. C., Frankenburg, F. R., & Fitzmaurice, G. M. (2013). Defense mechanisms reported by patients with borderline personality disorder and axis II comparison subjects over 16 years of prospective follow-up: Description and prediction of recovery. *American Journal of Psychiatry, 170,* 111–120.

Zanarini, M. C., Frankenburg, F. R., & Fitzmaurice, G. M. (2014). Severity of anxiety symptoms reported by borderline patients and axis II comparison subjects: Description and prediction over 16 years of prospective follow-up. *Journal of Personality Disorders, 28,* 767–777.

Zanarini, M. C., Frankenburg, F. R., Hennen, J., & Silk, K. R. (2003). The longitudinal course of borderline psychopathology: 6-year prospective follow-up of the phenomenology of borderline personality disorder. *American Journal of Psychiatry, 160,* 274–283.

Zanarini, M. C., Frankenburg, F. R., Hennen, J., & Silk, K. R. (2004). Mental health service utilization of borderline patients and axis II comparison subjects followed prospectively for six years. *Journal of Clinical Psychiatry, 65,* 28–36.

Zanarini, M. C., Frankenburg, F. R., Hennen, J., Reich, D. B., & Silk, K. R. (2004). Axis I comorbidity in patients with borderline personality disorder: 6-year follow-up and prediction of time to remission. *American Journal Psychiatry, 161,* 2108–2114.

Zanarini, M. C., Frankenburg, F. R., Hennen, J., Reich, D. B., & Silk, K. R. (2005). Psychosocial functioning of borderline patients and axis II comparison subjects followed prospectively for six years. *Journal of Personality Disorders, 19,* 19–29.

Zanarini, M. C., Frankenburg, F. R., Hennen, J., Reich, D. B., & Silk, K. R. (2006). Prediction of the 10-year course of borderline personality disorder. *American Journal of Psychiatry, 163,* 827–832.

Zanarini, M. C., Frankenburg, F. R., Jager-Hyman, S., Reich, D. B., & Fitzmaurice, G. M. (2008). The course of dissociation for patients with borderline personality disorder and axis II comparison subjects: A 10-year follow-up study. *Acta Psychiatrica Scandinavica, 118,* 291–296.

Zanarini, M. C., Frankenburg, F. R., Khera, G. S., & Bleichmar, J. (2001). Treatment histories of borderline inpatients. *Comprehensive Psychiatry, 42,* 144–150.

Zanarini, M. C., Frankenburg, F. R., Marino, M. F., Reich, D. B., Haynes, M. C., & Gunderson, J. G. (1999). Violence in the lives of adult borderline patients. *Journal of Nervous and Mental Disease, 187,* 65–71.

Zanarini, M. C., Frankenburg, F. R., & Parachini, E. A. (2004). A preliminary, randomized trial of fluoxetine, olanzapine, and the olanzapine-fluoxetine combination in women with borderline personality disorder. *Journal of Clinical Psychiatry, 65*, 903–907.

Zanarini, M. C., Frankenburg, F. R., Reich, D. B., Conkey, L. C., & Fitzmaurice, G. M. (2015). Treatment rates for patients with borderline personality disorder and other personality disorders: A 16-year study. *Psychiatric Services, 66*, 15–20.

Zanarini, M. C., Frankenburg, F. R., Reich, D. B., & Fitzmaurice, G. M. (2010a). The 10-year course of psychosocial functioning among patients with borderline personality disorder and axis II comparison subjects. *Acta Psychiatrica Scandinavica, 122*, 103–109.

Zanarini, M. C., Frankenburg, F. R., Reich, D. B., & Fitzmaurice, G. M. (2010b). Time-to-attainment of recovery from borderline personality disorder and its stability: A 10-year prospective follow-up study. *American Journal of Psychiatry, 167*, 663–667.

Zanarini, M. C., Frankenburg, F. R., Reich, D. B., & Fitzmaurice, G. M. (2012). Attainment and stability of sustained symptomatic remission and recovery among borderline patients and axis II comparison subjects: A 16-year prospective follow-up study. *American Journal of Psychiatry, 169*, 476–483.

Zanarini, M. C., Frankenburg, F. R., Reich, D. B., & Fitzmaurice, G. M. (2016). Fluidity of the subsyndromal phenomenology of borderline personality disorder over 16 years of prospective follow-up. *American Journal of Psychiatry, 173*, 688–694.

Zanarini, M. C., Frankenburg, F. R., Reich, D. B., Fitzmaurice, G. M., Weinberg, I., & Gunderson, J. G. (2008). 10-year course of physically self-destructive acts reported by borderline patients and axis II comparison subjects. *Acta Psychiatrica Scandinavica, 117*, 177–184.

Zanarini, M. C., Frankenburg, F. R., Reich, B. D., Harned, A. L., & Fitzmaurice, G. M. (2015). Rates of psychotropic medication use reported by borderline patients and axis II comparison subjects over 16 years of prospective follow-up. *Journal of Clinical Psychopharmacology, 35*, 63–67.

Zanarini, M. C., Frankenburg, F. R., Reich, D. B., Hennen, J., & Silk, K. R. (2005). Adult experiences of abuse reported by borderline patients and axis II comparison subjects over six years of prospective follow-up. *Journal of Nervous and Mental Disease, 193*, 412–416.

Zanarini, M. C., Frankenburg, F. R., Reich, D. B., Marino, M. F., Lewis, R. E., Williams, A. A., & Khera, G. S. (2000). Biparental failure in the childhood experiences of borderline patients. *Journal of Personality Disorders, 14*, 264–273.

Zanarini, M. C., Frankenburg, F. R., Reich, D. B., Silk, K. R., Hudson, J. I., & McSweeney, L. B. (2007). The subsyndromal phenomenology of borderline personality disorder: A 10-year follow-up study. *American Journal of Psychiatry, 164*, 929–935.

Zanarini, M. C., Frankenburg, F. R., Reich, D. B., Wedig, M. M., Conkey, L. C., & Fitzmaurice GM. (2014). Prediction of time-to-attainment of recovery for borderline patients followed prospectively for 16 years. *Acta Psychiatrica Scandinavica, 130*, 205–213.

Zanarini, M. C., Frankenburg, F. R., Reich, D. B., Wedig, M. M., Conkey, L. C., & Fitzmaurice, G. M. (2015). The course of marriage/sustained cohabitation and parenthood among borderline patients followed prospectively for 16 years. *Journal of Personality Disorders, 29*, 62–70.

Zanarini, M. C., Frankenburg, F. R., Ridolfi, M. E., Jager-Hyman, S., Hennen, J., & Gunderson, J. G. (2006). Reported childhood onset to self-mutilation among borderline patients. *Journal of Personality Disorders, 20,* 9–15.

Zanarini, M. C., Frankenburg, F. R., & Vujanovic, A. A. (2002). The interrater and test-retest reliability of the Revised Diagnostic Interview for Borderlines (DIB-R). *Journal of Personality Disorders, 16,* 270–276.

Zanarini, M. C., Frankenburg, F. R., Vujanovic, A. A., Hennen, J., Reich, D. B., & Silk, K. R. (2004). Axis II comorbidity of borderline personality disorder: Description of six-year course and prediction to time-to-remission. *Acta Psychiatrica Scandinavica, 110,* 416–420.

Zanarini, M. C., Frankenburg, F. R., Wedig, M. M., & Fitzmaurice, G. M. (2013). Cognitive experiences reported by borderline patients and axis II comparison subjects: A 16-year prospective follow-up study. *American Journal Psychiatry, 170,* 671–679.

Zanarini, M. C., Frankenburg, F. R., Weingeroff, J. L., Reich, D. B., Fitzmaurice, G. M., & Weiss, R. D. (2011). The course of substance use disorders in patients with borderline personality disorder and axis II comparison subjects: A 10-year follow-up study. *Addiction, 106,* 342–348.

Zanarini, M. C., Frankenburg, F. R., Yong, L., Raviola, G., Reich, D. B., Hennen, J., & Gunderson, J. G. (2004). Borderline psychopathology in the first-degree relatives of borderline and axis II comparison probands. *Journal of Personality Disorders, 18,* 439–447.

Zanarini, M. C., Gunderson, J. G., & Frankenburg, F. R. (1990). Cognitive features of borderline personality disorder. *American Journal Psychiatry, 147,* 57–63.

Zanarini, M. C., Gunderson, J. G., Frankenburg, F. R., & Chauncey, D. L. (1989). The revised diagnostic interview for borderlines: Discriminating BPD from other axis II disorders. *Journal of Personality Disorders, 3,* 10–18.

Zanarini, M. C., Gunderson, J. G., Frankenburg, F. R., & Chauncey, D. L. (1990). Discriminating borderline personality disorder from other axis II disorders. *American Journal of Psychiatry, 147,* 161–167.

Zanarini, M. C., Gunderson, J. G., Marino, M. F., Schwartz, E. O., & Frankenburg, F. R. (1988). DSM-III disorders in the families of borderline outpatients. *Journal of Personality Disorders, 2,* 292–302.

Zanarini, M. C., Gunderson, J. G., Marino, M. F., Schwartz, E. O., & Frankenburg, F. R. (1989). Childhood experiences of borderline patients. *Comprehensive Psychiatry, 30,* 18–25.

Zanarini, M. C., Hörz-Sagstetter, S., Frankenburg, F. R., Reich, D. B., & Fitzmaurice, G. M. (Under review). The 16-year course of major depression and bipolar disorder in patients with borderline personality disorder and axis II comparison subjects.

Zanarini, M. C., Hörz, S., Frankenburg, F. R., Weingeroff, J., Reich, D. B., & Fitzmaurice, G. M. (2011). The 10-year course of PTSD in borderline patients and axis II comparison subjects. *Acta Psychiatrica Scandinavica, 124,* 349–356.

Zanarini, M. C., Jacoby, R. J., Frankenburg, F. R., Reich, D. B., & Fitzmaurice, G. M. (2009). The 10-year course of Social Security disability income reported by

borderline patients and axis II comparison subjects. *Journal of Personality Disorders,*
23, 346–356.

Zanarini, M. C., Laudate, C. S., Frankenburg, F. R., Reich, D. B., & Fitzmaurice, G. M.
(2011). Predictors of self-mutilation in patients with borderline personality disorder: A 10-year follow-up study. *Journal of Psychiatric Research, 45,* 823–828.

Zanarini, M. C., Laudate, C. S., Frankenburg, F. R., Wedig, M. M., & Fitzmaurice, G. M.
(2013). Reasons for self-mutilation reported by borderline patients over 16 years of
prospective follow-up. *Journal of Personality Disorders, 27,* 783–794.

Zanarini, M. C., Parachini, E. A., Frankenburg, F. R., Holman, J. B., Hennen, J., Reich, D.
B., & Silk, K. R. (2003). Sexual relationship difficulties among borderline patients and
axis II comparison subjects. *Journal of Nervous and Mental Disease, 191,*479–482.

Zanarini, M. C., Reichman, C. A., Frankenburg, F. R., Reich, D. B., & Fitzmaurice, G.
M. (2010). The course of eating disorders in patients with borderline personality disorder: A 10-year follow-up study. *International Journal Eating Disorders, 43,* 226–232.

Zanarini, M. C., Ruser, T., Frankenburg, F. R., & Hennen, J. (2000). The dissociative
experiences of borderline patients. *Comprehensive Psychiatry, 41,* 223–227.

Zanarini, M. C., Ruser, T., Frankenburg, F. R., Hennen, J., & Gunderson, J. G. (2000).
Risk factors associated with the dissociative experiences of borderline patients.
Journal of Nervous and Mental Disease, 188, 26–30.

Zanarini, M. C., Schulz, S. C., Detke, H. C., Tanaka, Y., Zhao, F., Lin, D., . . . Corya, S.
(2011). A dose comparison of olanzapine for the treatment of borderline personality
disorder: A 12-week randomized, double-blind, placebo-controlled study. *Journal of*
Clinical Psychiatry, 72, 1353–1362.

Zanarini, M. C., Weingeroff, J., & Frankenburg, F. R. (2009). Defense mechanisms associated with borderline personality disorder. *Journal of Personality Disorders, 23,*
113–121.

Zanarini, M. C., Williams, A. A., Lewis, R. E., Reich, D. B., Vera, S. C., Marino, M.
F., . . . Frankenburg, F. R. (1997). Reported pathological childhood experiences asso-
ciated with the development of borderline personality disorder. *American Journal of*
Psychiatry, 154, 1101–1111.

Zanarini, M. C., Yong, L., Frankenburg, F. R., Hennen, J., Reich, D. B., & Marino, M.
(2002). Severity of reported childhood sexual abuse and its relationship to severity
of borderline psychopathology and psychosocial impairment. *Journal of Nervous and*
Mental Disease, 190, 381–387.

Zetzel, E. R. (1968). The so-called good hysteric. *International Journal of Psychoanalysis,*
49, 256–260.

Zilboorg, G. (1941). Ambulatory schizophrenia. *Psychiatry, 4,* 149–155.

Zittel Conklin, C., & Westen, D. (2005). Borderline personality disorder in clinical practice. *American Journal of Psychiatry, 162,* 867–875.

Zweig-Frank, H., Paris, J., & Guzder, J. (1994a). Dissociation in female patients with
borderline and non-borderline personality disorders. *Journal Personality Disorders,*
8, 203–209.

Zweig-Frank, H., Paris, J., & Guzder, J. (1994b). Dissociation in male patients with
borderline and non-borderline personality disorders. *Journal Personality Disorders,*
8, 210–218.

Mary C. Zanarini, EdD, is a professor of psychology at Harvard Medical School and director of McLean Hospital's Laboratory for the Study of Adult Development. She has spent her career studying the phenomenology and long-term course of borderline personality disorder (BPD), childhood experiences of adversity, and co-occurring disorders. She has also conducted a series of medication trials and trials of psychosocial treatments for BPD. In addition, she developed the most widely used diagnostic and severity measures for BPD. Dr. Zanarini is the founding president of the North American Society for the Study of Personality Disorders, has won numerous awards, and has had her work funded by a number of sources (NIMH, NARSAD, American Foundation for Suicide Prevention, and the Templeton Foundation).

abandonment concerns, 12–13, 70, 92–93

absorption, 42

abuse

adult victimization, risk factor
for, 172–73

anxiety prediction, 100

in childhood, studies of, 14

McLean Study of Adult Development
findings, 40–41

self-mutilation prediction, 89, 90

shame prediction, 101–2

acting out, 184–86

acute symptoms

general discussion, 70–71

sixteen-year follow-up, 74–77

ten-year follow-up, 72–74

Adler, G., 12

adult victimization

baseline findings, 171–72

overview, 171

self-mutilation prediction, 89

by six-year follow-up, 172–73

suicide attempt prediction, 94

by ten-year follow-up, 173–74

time-to-recovery prediction, 139

adverse childhood experiences. *See*
childhood adversity

affective reasons for self-mutilation, 91

affective spectrum disorder, 5

affective symptoms, 69

follow-up studies, 72–74

over time, 99

predictor of suicide attempts, 94

agoraphobia, 146–47

agreeableness, 131, 138

Akiskal, H. S., 24

alcohol abuse, 25, 53–54, 144–45

aloneness, intolerance of, 70

ambulatory schizophrenia, 3

amnesia, 42

anorexia, 145

anticonvulsants, 156

antidepressants, 156

Antikainen, R., 27

antipsychotics, 156

antisocial personality disorder
(APD), 24–25

anxiety, 99–100

anxiety disorders, 41–42

by six-year follow-up, 141–42

by ten-year follow-up, 144, 146–47

anxiolytics, 156

anxious cluster personality disorders,
138, 143

APD (antisocial personality
disorder), 24–25

avoidant personality disorder, 143

Axis I disorders

by six-year follow-up, 141–42

by ten-year follow-up, 144

Axis II disorders, by six-year
follow-up, 143

Barasch, A., 24

Baseline Information Schedule
    (BIS), 43–44

Bateman, A., 75

BED (binge eating disorder), 145

behavioral strategies, 11, 18–20

benzodiazepines, 156

binge eating disorder (BED), 145

biological dysfunction, 48

bipolar disorder
  by sixteen-year follow-up, 147–48
  treatments based on, 6

BIS (Baseline Information
    Schedule), 43–44

bisexual orientation, 178–79

body mass index (BMI), 163–64

Bond, M., 181–82

borderline defenses, 182–84, 185–86

borderline personality organization
    (BPO), 4

boundaries, teaching, 63

BPDPSYCHOED program, 86

BPO (borderline personality
    organization), 4

Buie, D., 12, 62

bulimia, 145

caretaker abuse and neglect
  adult victimization, risk factor
    for, 172–74
  self-mutilation and, 90
  shame prediction, 101–2
  studies of, 15, 40–41

Carpenter, W. T., 33–34

CBMI (cumulative body mass
    index), 164–65

childhood adversity
  adult victimization, risk factor
    for, 172–74
  anxiety prediction, 100
  current knowledge concerning, 16
  empirical investigations of, 13–15
  McLean Study of Adult
    Development, 40–41
  psychoanalytic theories of
    pathogenesis, 12

recovery prediction, 133–34

self-mutilation prediction, 89, 90

shame prediction, 101–2

time-to-recovery prediction, 139

tripartite model of etiology, 8

chronic medical conditions, 161–63

Clarkin, J., 16–17, 24, 75

CLPS. See Collaborative Longitudinal
    Personality Disorders Study

cognitive reasons for self-mutilation, 91

cognitive symptoms, 49–50
  assessed by DIB-R in sixteen-year
    follow-up, 105
  follow-up studies, 70, 72–74
  over time, 102–4

Collaborative Longitudinal Personality
    Disorders Study (CLPS), 33–34
  mental health treatment, 157–58
  psychosocial functioning, 114–15
  recovery, 121–22
  remission, 85
  symptoms over time, 76–77

complex comorbidity, 142–43

complex model of borderline
    psychopathology, 8–9, 20

continuum of borderline
    psychopathology, 9–10

convergent validity of psychosocial
    functioning, 39–40

co-occurring disorders
  anxiety disorders by ten-year
    follow-up, 146–47
  Axis I disorders, 141–42, 144
  Axis II disorders, 143
  continuum of borderline
    psychopathology, 10
  eating disorders, 145
  McLean Study of Adult
    Development, 41–42
  mood disorders, 147–48
  PTSD, 146
  short-term studies
    from 1980s, 23–26
    from 1990s, 26–28
  substance use disorders, 144–45
  suicide attempt prediction, 94

Cooper, S., 24–25
counterdependency, 63–64, 70
countertransference problems, 70, 71
cumulative body mass index (CBMI),
    164–65

DBAS-16 (Dysfunctional Beliefs
    and Attitudes about Sleep
    questionnaire), 166–67
DBT (dialectical behavioral therapy), 27
deaths
    of other causes, 96
    by suicide, 94–96
defense mechanisms
    cross-sectional baseline data
        on, 182–85
    overview, 181
    by sixteen-year follow-up, 185–87
    study of, 181–82
Defense Style Questionnaire, 181–82
delusions, 49–50, 70
demandingness
    follow-up studies, 70
    general discussion, 58
    suicide threby prediction, 92–93
dependency, 63–64, 70
dependent personality disorder, 143
depression
    by sixteen-year follow-up, 147–48
    suicidality, 53–55
    suicide attempt prediction, 94
DES (Dissociative Experiences Scale),
    42, 102–4
determination, 190
Deutsch, H., 3
devaluation, 56, 70
diagnosis, reluctance to give, 1–2
*Diagnostic and Statistical Manual of
    Mental Disorders* (*DSM*)
    cognitive symptoms in, 106
    DSM-III-R criteria for BPD, 45–46, 106
Diagnostic Interview for Borderlines
    (DIB), 25
dialectical behavioral therapy (DBT), 27
DIB-R (Revised Diagnostic Interview for
    Borderlines), 45, 46–47, 105

disability, 108–9, 110–12, 113
dissociation, 42, 89
    over time, 102–4
    predictor of suicide attempts, 94
Dissociative Experiences Scale (DES),
    42, 102–4
distortions of truth, 64–65
disturbed parental involvement, 14
DSM. See *Diagnostic and Statistical
    Manual of Mental Disorders*
Dysfunctional Beliefs and Attitudes
    about Sleep questionnaire
    (DBAS-16), 166–67
dysphoria, 48–49
    follow-up studies, 73–74
    persistence of, 69
    self-mutilation and, 89–90

early separations and losses, 13–14
eating disorder not otherwise specified
    (EDNOS), 145
eating disorders, 41–42
    by six-year follow-up, 141–42
    by ten-year follow-up, 144, 145
emotional abuse
    adult victimization, 172–74
    in childhood, 14, 100, 101–2
emotional hypochondriasis,
    184–86
emotional neglect in childhood, 15
empirical investigations of environmental
    factors, 13–15
entitlement, 59, 70
environmental factors, 12–13
    empirical investigations of, 13–15
    psychoanalytic theories of
        pathogenesis, 12
etiology
    of behavioral and interpersonal
        strategies, 18–20
    environmental factors, 12–13
    of inner pain, 16–17
    tripartite model of, 8
exercise
    by sixteen-year follow-up, 163
    by six-year follow-up, 161–62

experiential avoidance, 190–91
extra-session contact, 63–64
extraversion, 138

Family Connections program, 86
family history of psychiatric disorder,
    18–19, 41, 139
family training programs, 86
fear of abandonment, 12–13
fighting spirit, 10
Fitzmaurice, G. M., 111
follow-back studies
  descriptions of, 29–32
  lessons learned from, 33
Fonagy, P., 75
Frances, A., 24
Frankenburg, F. R., 8–9, 107, 111,
    114, 143
Freud, A., 181
friendships with therapists, 62
Frosch, J., 3–4

GAD (generalized anxiety
    disorder), 146–47
GAF (Global Assessment of Functioning),
    31, 121–22
GAS (Global Assessment Score),
    24–25, 121
gender of relationship choice, 178–79
generalized anxiety disorder
    (GAD), 146–47
Giesen-Bloo, J., 75
Global Assessment of Functioning (GAF),
    31, 121–22
Global Assessment Score (GAS),
    24–25, 121
Grinker, R. R., 32
grit, 190
group therapies, 149–50
guilt, overvalued ideas of, 49–50
Gunderson, J. G., 4–5, 7, 23, 28, 33–34, 77,
    85, 121

hallucinations, 49–50, 70
health. See physical health

Health Sickness Rating Scale (HSRS), 27
Heard, H. L., 27
Hennen, J., 8–9, 107
heritability, 18–19, 140
Herman, J. L., 5, 171
history of disorder
  other terms used for, 3
  place in psychiatric nomenclature, 5–6
  schizophrenia, linked to, 3
  work of Gunderson and Singer, 4–5
  work of Kernberg, 4
  work of Stern, 2
Hoch, P. H., 3
homosexual orientation, 178–79
hopelessness, 92–93
hospitalization
  CLPS study results, 157–58
  prediction of time-to-recovery, 137–38
  short-term studies
    from 1960s-1970s, 21–22
    from 1980s, 23–26
    from 1990s, 26–28
  by sixteen-year follow-up, 155
  by six-year follow up, 152–53
  by ten-year follow-up, 154
HSRS (Health Sickness Rating Scale), 27
Hudson, J. I., 23
humor, 186
Hurt, S., 24
hyperbolic temperament, 8–9, 16–17, 48
hypersensitivity, 2–3

IBS (irritable bowel syndrome), 168–69
image-distorting defenses, 182–84, 185–86
immature defenses, 181–84, 185–86
impulse spectrum disorder, 5
impulsive action patterns, 11, 18–20
impulsive symptoms. See also self-
    mutilation; suicidality
  follow-up studies, 72–74
  remission of, 69–70
inferiority, feelings of, 2–3
inner pain
  etiology of, 16–17
  prevalence of, 42

self-defeating manner of handling, 11
   severity of, 11
inpatient staff, treatment regressions
      triggered by, 61
intelligence, in time-to-recovery
      prediction, 138, 139
intensive polypharmacy, 152–53
interpersonal reasons for
      self-mutilation, 91
interpersonal strategies, etiology of, 18–20
interpersonal symptoms
   demandingness, 58, 70, 92–93
   devaluation, 56, 70
   entitlement, 59, 70
   follow-up studies, 70, 72–74
   manipulation, 57, 70, 92–93
inter-rater reliability, 39
intimate partner violence, 171–72
intimate relationships
   gender of relationship choice, 178–79
   sexual relationship difficulties, 175–77
   by sixteen-year follow-up, 115–16
   by six-year follow-up, 107–11
   by ten-year follow-up, 111–15
IQ, in time-to-recovery prediction, 138
irritable bowel syndrome (IBS), 168–69

Jacoby, R. J., 111

Kernberg, O. F., 4, 12, 181–82
kindling events, 8–9
   empirical investigations of, 13–15
   normative nature of, 17–18
Knight, R. P., 3

Lenzenweger, M. F., 75
Levy, K. N., 75
lifestyle choices
   by sixteen-year follow-up, 163
   by six-year follow-up, 161–62
lifetime histories of psychiatric
      treatment, 150–51
Linehan, M. M., 7, 27
Links, P. S., 5, 26, 112
lithium, 156

longitudinal course studies
   follow-back studies, 29–33
   overview, 21
   prospective studies
      from 1960s-1970s, 21–22
      from 1980s, 23–26
      from 1990s, 26–28
      lessons learned from, 28
      overview, 21
long-term course of symptoms
   recurrence, 83–86
   remission, 81–83
   by sixteen-year follow-up, 74–77
   by six-year follow-up, 67–71
   by ten-year follow-up, 72–74
losses, early, 13–14
love affairs with therapists, 62

Maltsberger, J., 62
manipulation
   follow-up studies, 70
   general discussion, 57
   predictors of suicide threat, 92–93
MAO (monoamine oxidase) inhibitor, 156
marriage
   sexual relationship difficulties, 175–77
   by sixteen-year follow-up, 115–16
   by six-year follow-up, 107–11
   by ten-year follow-up, 111–15
masochism, 2–3, 65, 70
Masterson, J., 12–13
mature defenses, 181–82, 185–86
McGlashan, T. H., 30, 77, 121, 133–34
McLean Study of Adult
      Development (MSAD)
   childhood adversity, 40–41
   convergent validity of psychosocial
      functioning, 39–40
   co-occurring disorders, 41–42
   dependency and
      counterdependency, 63–64
   distortions of truth, 64–65
   family history of psychiatric disorder, 41
   prospective assessment over time, 43–44
   reliability sub-studies, 38–39

McLean Study of Adult
	Development (MSAD) (*cont.*)
	research design and measures, 35–37
	sadomasochistic tendencies, 65
	sample retention, 38
	sectors of psychopathology studied, 36
	self-mutilation, onset of, 42–43
	sixteen-year follow-up, 74–77
	six-year follow-up, 67–71
	special relationships, 62
	study criteria sets, 45–47
	subjects, 37
	subsyndromal phenomenology, 42
	ten-year follow-up, 72–74
	treatment history prior to study
		entry, 43
	treatment regressions, 60–61
McMain, S. F., 75
Meares, R., 27
medical conditions, chronic, 161–63
Mehlum, L., 27
mental health treatment
	CLPS study results, 157–58
	history prior to study entry, 43
	lifetime histories of psychiatric
		treatment, 150–51
	McLean Study of Adult
		Development, 43
	overview, 149–50
	psychiatric hospitalizations, 159
	psychotherapy, 158
	psychotropic medication, 156, 158
	by sixteen-year follow-up, 155
	by six-year follow-up, 152–54
	by ten-year follow-up, 154
models of borderline psychopathology
	attachment disorder, 7
	complex model, 8–9
	continuum of borderline
		psychopathology, 9–10
	emotional dysregulation, 7
	key features of disorder, 11
	tripartite model of etiology, 8
Modestin, J., 26, 112
monoamine oxidase (MAO) inhibitor, 156

mood disorders, 23–24, 41–42, 53–54
	remission and recurrence of BPD
		compared to, 85
	by sixteen-year follow-up, 147–48
	by six-year follow-up, 141–42
mood stabilizers, 156
more-intensive treatment, 153–54
Morey, L. C., 16–17
mothering, failures in, 12
MSAD. *See* McLean Study of Adult
		Development

Nace, E. P., 25
Najavits, L. M., 28
narcissistic character traits, 2–3
National Educational Alliance for
		Borderline Personality Disorder
		(NEA-BPD), 86
negative therapeutic reactions, 2–3
neglect in childhood
	adult victimization, risk factor
		for, 172–74
	self-mutilation and, 90
	shame prediction, 101–2
	studies of, 15, 40–41
neurotic defenses, 181–82, 185–86
neuroticism, 131
non-delusional paranoia, 105

obesity, 158–59, 163–64
obsessive-compulsive disorder
		(OCD), 146–47
odd thinking, 105
opioid medication, 168
outmoded survival strategies, 11, 93–94
outpatient treatment, 153–54
overvalued ideas of worthlessness and
		guilt, 49–50

pain, inner. *See* inner pain
pain, physical, 167–68
panic disorder, 146–47
paranoia, non-delusional, 105
parental involvement, disturbed, 14
parenthood

by sixteen-year follow-up, 115–16
by six-year follow-up, 108
Paris, J., 31, 133–34
Perry, J., 24–25
physical abuse
   adult victimization, 172–74
   in childhood, 14–15, 40–41
physical health
   irritable bowel syndrome, 168–69
   obesity and related conditions, 163–64
   pain, 167–68
   psychotropic medication, weight gain
      from, 158–59
   by sixteen-year follow-up, 163
   by six-year follow-up, 161–62
   sleep disturbances, 165–67
physical neglect in childhood, studies of, 15
Pittsburgh Sleep Quality Index
      (PSQI), 165–66
Plakun, E. M., 29, 133–34
Polatin, P., 3
Pope, H. G., 23
post-traumatic stress disorder (PTSD), 5
   predictor of suicide attempts, 94
   risk factor for obesity, 164
   by six-year follow-up, 141–42
   by ten-year follow-up, 144, 146
prediction of recovery from BPD, 133–40
prediction of remission of BPD, 130–33
prognosis, 85–86
projection, 186
projective defenses, 2–3
prospective studies
   from 1960s-1970s, 21–22
   from 1980s, 23–26
   from 1990s, 26–28
   lessons learned from, 28
   McLean Study of Adult
      Development, 43–44
   overview, 21
pseudoneurotic schizophrenia, 3
PSQI (Pittsburgh Sleep Quality
      Index), 165–66
psychiatric hospitalizations. See
   hospitalization

psychiatric treatment. See mental health
   treatment
psychic bleeding, 2–3
psychic rigidity, 2–3
psychoanalytic theories of pathogenesis, 12
psychoeducation program, 86
psychosocial functioning, 10
   convergent validity of, in MSAD,
      39–40
   overview, 107
   prediction of time-to-remission, 130
   short-term studies
      from 1960s-1970s, 21–22
      from 1980s, 23–26
      from 1990s, 26–28
   by sixteen-year follow-up, 115–16
   by six-year follow-up, 107–11
   by ten-year follow-up, 111–15
psychotherapy
   CLPS study results, 157–58
   general discussion, 158
   recommended, 149–50
   by sixteen-year follow-up, 155
   by six-year follow up, 152–53
   by ten-year follow-up, 154
psychotic character, 3–4
psychotic-like symptoms, 49–51, 70,
      71, 105
psychotropic medications
   CLPS study results, 157–58
   general discussion, 158
   overview, 150
   by sixteen-year follow-up, 155, 156
   by six-year follow up, 152–53
   by ten-year follow-up, 154
PTSD. See post-traumatic stress disorder

quasi-psychotic thought, 49–51, 70, 71, 105

rape, 171–72, 175–77
reality-testing, 2–3
recovery, 190–91
   attitude towards, 10
   comparing with other follow-up
      studies, 121

recovery, (*cont.*)
  cumulative rates of, 118–20
  defining, 117
  heritability of interpersonal factors, 140
  sleep quality and, 165–67
  time-to-recovery predictions, 133–40
recurrence
  general discussion, 83–86
  sixteen-year follow-up study, 74–77
regressions, treatment, 60–61
Reich, D. B., 8–9, 111, 115
relationships with therapists, 62
reliability sub-studies, 38–39
remission of symptoms
  by sixteen-year follow-up, 74–77
  by ten-year follow-up, 72–74
research design and measures, 35–37
resilience, 190–91
retrospective studies
  descriptions of, 29–32
  lessons learned from, 33
Revised Diagnostic Interview for
     Borderlines (DIB-R), 45,
     46–47, 105
romantic relationships
  gender of relationship choice, 178–79
  love affairs with therapists, 62
  sexual relationship difficulties, 175–77

sadism, 65, 70
sample retention, 38
Sandell, R., 27, 112
schizophrenia, disorder historically
     linked to, 3
Schmideberg, M., 3
selective serotonin reuptake inhibitor
     (SSRI), 156
self-defeating personality disorder, 143
self-mutilation
  behavioral strategies, etiology of, 18–20
  general discussion, 51–52
  McLean Study of Adult
     Development, 42–43
  predictors of, 87–90
  prevalence of, 69–70

reasons for, 87–91
suicide attempt prediction, 94
self-report instruments, 36–37
semi-structured interviews, 35–37
Senol, S., 28
separations, early, 13–14, 41
sexual abuse
  adult victimization, risk factor
     for, 172–74
  McLean Study of Adult
     Development, 40–41
  self-mutilation prediction, 89
  sexual relationship difficulties due
     to, 175–77
  shame prediction, 101–2
  studies of, 14–15
  time-to-recovery prediction, 136–37
sexual issues
  gender of relationship choice, 178–79
  overview, 175
  sexual orientation, 178–79
  sexual relationship difficulties, 175–77
shame, 101–2
Shea, M. T., 76–77
short-term studies
  from 1960s–1970s, 21–22
  from 1980s, 23–26
  from 1990s, 26–28
  lessons learned from, 28
  overview, 21
Silk, K. R., 8–9
Singer, M. T., 4–5
sixteen-year follow-up
  cognitive symptoms, 105
  defense mechanisms, 185–87
  mental health treatment, 155
  mood disorders, 147–48
  physical health, 163
  psychosocial functioning, 115–16
  sexual relationship difficulties, 177
  symptoms, 74–77
six-year follow-up
  adult victimization, 172–73
  Axis I disorders, 141–42
  Axis II disorders, 143

mental health treatment, 152–54
physical health, 161–62
psychosocial functioning, 107–11
sexual relationship difficulties, 175–77
symptoms, 67–71
Skodol, A. E., 115
sleep disturbances, 165–67
social functioning
overview, 107
by sixteen-year follow-up, 115–16
by six-year follow-up, 107–11
by ten-year follow-up, 111–15
social phobia, 146–47
Social Security Disability Income (SSDI)
benefits, 111–12, 113
somatic insecurity or anxiety, 2–3
special relationships, 62
SSDI (Social Security Disability Income)
benefits, 111–12, 113
SSRI (selective serotonin reuptake
inhibitor), 156
STEPPS (systems training for emotional
predictability and problem
solving), 150
Stern, A., 2
Stevenson, J., 27
stigma related to diagnosis, 1–2
Stone, M. H., 32, 121, 133–34
Strauss, J. S., 33
subjects, in McLean Study of Adult
Development, 37
substance abuse, 53–54, 69–70, 94
substance use disorders (SUDs), 41–42
by six-year follow-up, 141–42
by ten-year follow-up, 144–45
subsyndromal phenomenology, 42
SUDs. See substance use disorders
suicidality
behavioral strategies, etiology
of, 18–20
general discussion, 53–55
predictors of attempts, 94
predictors of threat, 92–93
rates of completed, 94–96
survival strategies, outmoded, 11, 93–94

symptoms. See also interpersonal
symptoms; recurrence; remission;
self-mutilation; suicidality
affects over time, 99
anxiety, 99–100
baseline to six-year follow-up, 67–71
chronic and intense dysphoria,
48–49
cognitions over time, 102–4
cognitive, 49–50
dependency and
counterdependency, 63–64
dissociation, 42, 89, 94, 102–4
distortions of truth, 64–65
DSM nomenclature, cognitive
symptoms in, 106
impulsive, 51–55
sadomasochistic tendencies, 65
shame, 101–2
special relationships, 62
specific cognitions in sixteen-year
follow-up, 105
study criteria sets, 45–47
treatment regressions, 60–61
systems training for emotional
predictability and problem solving
(STEPPS), 150

temperamental predictors
of recovery, 138
of remission, 129
temperamental symptoms
general discussion, 70–71
sixteen-year follow-up, 74–77
ten-year follow-up, 72–74
ten-year follow-up
adult victimization, 173–74
anxiety disorders, 146–47
Axis I disorders, 144
eating disorders, 145
mental health treatment, 154
psychosocial functioning, 111–15
PTSD, 146
substance use disorders, 144–45
symptoms, 72–74

therapists
  dependency on, 63–64
  sadomasochistic tendencies,
    handling, 65
  special relationships with, 62
  translation process, 56–57
time-to-cessation of treatment, 154
time-to-recovery prediction, 133–40
time-to-remission prediction, 130–33
time-to-resumption of treatment, 154
translation process, 56–57
treatment. *See* mental health treatment
treatment regressions
  follow-up studies, 70
  general discussion, 60–61
  resolution of, 71
tricyclic antidepressants, 156
triggering events. *See* kindling events
tripartite model of etiology, 8
true-psychotic thought, 105
truth, distortions of, 64–65
Tucker, L., 25

undoing, 184–86
unusual perceptual experiences, 105

Vaillant, G. E., 63, 181–82
Van Der Kolk, B. A., 5, 171

verbal abuse
  adult victimization, 172–74
  in childhood
    anxiety prediction, 100
    shame prediction, 101–2
    studies of, 14, 40–41
Villiger, C., 26, 112
vocational counseling, 113
vocational functioning
  overview, 107
  prediction of time-to-recovery, 138
  by sixteen-year follow-up, 115–16
  by six-year follow-up, 107–11
  by ten-year follow-up, 111–15
voice mail, 64
Vujanovic, A. A., 143
vulnerable temperament, 8–9, 16–17

Wedig, M. M., 115
Werble, B., 33
work. *See* vocational functioning
worthlessness, overvalued ideas of, 49–50

Zanarini, M. C., 8–9, 107, 111,
  115, 143
Zetzel, E. R., 3
Zilboorg, G., 3
Zweig-Frank, H., 31